FOOTBALL SHORT STORIES FOR KIDS

Charlotte Gibbs

© Copyright 2023 - All rights reserved.

The content contained within this book may not be reproduced, duplicated or transmitted without direct written permission from the author or the publisher.

Under no circumstances will any blame or legal responsibility be held against the publisher, or author, for any damages, reparation, or monetary loss due to the information contained within this book, either directly or indirectly.

Legal Notice:

This book is copyright protected. It is only for personal use. You cannot amend, distribute, sell, use, quote or paraphrase any part, or the content within this book, without the consent of the author or publisher.

Disclaimer Notice:

Please note the information contained within this document is for educational and entertainment purposes only. All effort has been executed to present accurate, up to date, reliable, complete information. No warranties of any kind are declared or implied. Readers acknowledge that the author is not engaged in the rendering of legal, financial, medical or professional advice. The content within this book has been derived from various sources. Please consult a licensed professional before attempting any techniques outlined in this book.

By reading this document, the reader agrees that under no circumstances is the author responsible for any losses, direct or indirect, that are incurred as a result of the use of the information contained within this document, including, but not limited to, errors, omissions, or inaccuracies.

TABLE OF CONTENTS

Introduction
6

CHAPTER 1
The Immaculate Reception
8

CHAPTER 2
The Fumble Fiasco
14

CHAPTER 3
The Rookie Sensation
19

CHAPTER 4
The Touchdown Celebration Extravaganza
25

CHAPTER 5
When You Wish
30

CHAPTER 6
The Legendary Quarterback
37

CHAPTER 7
The Football Magician
42

CHAPTER 8
The Beauty of Beast Mode
47

CHAPTER 9
Philly, Philly—Oh, so Special!
51

CHAPTER 10
The Comeback Kings
55

CHAPTER 11
The MVP Siblings
60

CHAPTER 12
The Super Bowl Surprise
65

CHAPTER 13
Megatron's Magical Hands
69

CHAPTER 14
A Swipe of the Brush after Dashes and Passes: Ernie Barnes
74

CHAPTER 15
Masters for Hurts
78

CHAPTER 16
A Perfect Miracle in Miami
84

CHAPTER 17
For #3, With Love
89

CHAPTER 18
The Icy (Ice) Bowl
94

CHAPTER 19
Jumpin' Lambeau, Lambeau Leap
98

CHAPTER 20
A Fail Mary—Which Call Should've Stood?
103

Conclusion
109

References
111

INTRODUCTION

Imagine a scenario where all eyes are on you. Thousands of fans are watching your every move, waiting for you to pass a touchdown or make an epic comeback to win the game. The once roaring crowds have gone eerily silent, eagerly awaiting your next move. Okay, okay—maybe you're not a professional athlete, but you're a human being just like these football stars. Whether it's a school project, worries, or making friends, we all feel the pressure from time to time. These American footballers show us that mistakes, funny mishaps and nail-biting moments are totally normal—they're just like us, who would've thought?.

The history of American football dates back to 1869, with its origin roots sourcing from the likes of soccer and rugby. The sport progressed at college level for many years to come and, in 1920, the first official National Football League (NFL) game was played and the rest is history.

From unforgettable football plays to hilarious viral moments, these short stories will inspire the young generation and teach you that it's okay if you fall down so long as you laugh, get back up, and try again.

Maybe you'll start thinking about a new creative solution to a problem, or perhaps you'll discover a passion for helping out others. Whatever it is, I'm sure it will add great value to your life.

Football Short Stories for Kids Touchdown Tales is an anthological collection of short stories by Charlotte Gibbs where the trials and tribulations of American Football are told to make you laugh, think, and learn something.

Isn't it great to know that our heroes aren't perfect either?

CHAPTER 1

THE IMMACULATE RECEPTION

Immaculate. What a mouthful, but such a special word. Maybe you're wondering what it means. It's like "awesome", "superb", "really cool", or something you are unlikely ever to see again. Right place, right time—that kind of thing. Fingertips ready, saving that pigskin from touching the field, some 60,000 people watching, and run, run, run away, getting closer, and whoop, there it is! A touchdown!

One of the most famous football plays of all time happened in December 1972; Pittsburgh Steelers against the Oakland Raiders. The Raiders were leading 7-6, the game was tight and fans were on edge, perhaps not so patiently waiting to see who would win. Football fans love to hate this famous moment because they argue if it was fair or if the Steelers just got lucky.

So, many questions—did the ball touch the ground before Steelers running back Franco Harris caught it?

Is the reason the referees didn't call the play dead because they couldn't see that his teammate, John Fuqua, perhaps deflected the ball?

Was it really "immaculate," or was it an "illegal double touch?"

With time ticking on the clock, tension and worry filled the air. Steelers quarterback Terry Bradshaw faced yet another tough choice; with no timeouts left, it looked like the tradition of never winning in the playoffs would continue for the Steelers.

Bradshaw steps back and throws on the fourth-and-10; the plays started on the Steelers' 40-yard line. What happens next is a true comedy of errors and missed calls, and fortunately for those Steeler fans, the instant replay wasn't invented yet! The final decision was always up to the judgment of the referee's own eyes. Oh, how times have changed.

The ball was possessed. No one could, at first, get a handle on the ball. Did it bounce off that helmet? It doesn't matter because Harris has scooped the ball just millimeters from the ground before taking off. What an unexpected twist.

And the question that had everyone on the edge of their seats; will he go all the way?

Ten yards turn to twenty, forty, then sixty yards. Harris was on a roll—he was unstoppable!

Yes!

Touchdown. Steelers!

The crowd is going wild. Cheers fill the air. The atmosphere was electric. A few worried about the huddled referees, and more anxious eyes focused on the refs. What were they discussing? More and more eyes were directed to the refs. Would they reverse the call?

Based on the rules back then, an offensive player couldn't catch a forward pass if another offensive player touched the ball beforehand. I guess it didn't help the refs because the ball seemed to have been bobbled and bounced around a bit, but the refs took their time and tried their best to make the right call. Moment after moment slowly went by. What would the refs do?

It kind of felt like one of those moments we're all familiar with. Time is passing slowly and each minute feels like it drags on for hours and hours. Everyone in that stadium was on edge, eagerly awaiting the final decision from the refs.

And then, after what felt like forever, they decided that the call on the field stood. It was a catch! Steelers fans were over the moon with the refs decision. Finally, the 1972 Steelers had a playoff victory under their belt.

What did (or should I say, can) we learn from the story of the Immaculate Reception? Sure, having things go perfectly is the best feeling, because it's easy to believe in yourself when things are working out for you. I also know it's hard to believe in yourself when things don't quite go your way and there are obstacles in the way, right? Of course it is, that's human nature. So, let's think back to the Steelers in that game; they could've given up, but they didnt—they were still pushing. They choose to have faith in their game, and in themselves, so much so that fate had to step in and lend a hand by allowing the ball to bounce the way it did for Harris to snatch it up and take it in for a touchdown (TD)!

Don't believe me? Think about it this way. How do you learn new things? You can wish all you want, but nothing really happens. When you ask for help or start practicing, things fall into place. The more you practice, the more your wishes come true because these wishes turn into having faith in yourself and your abilities. Whatever your goals are, if you mix belief and action, who knows what you can become. Whether it's a football player, a teacher, owning your own social media brand, or being the best kid you can be! With that balanced combination of belief and action, the world is your oyster. When you believe, success is so much easier to achieve. Don't overthink about your fears and doubts; don't let negative thoughts live in your mind. Remember, the lesson here is that greatness is inside you, and belief helps it to grow.

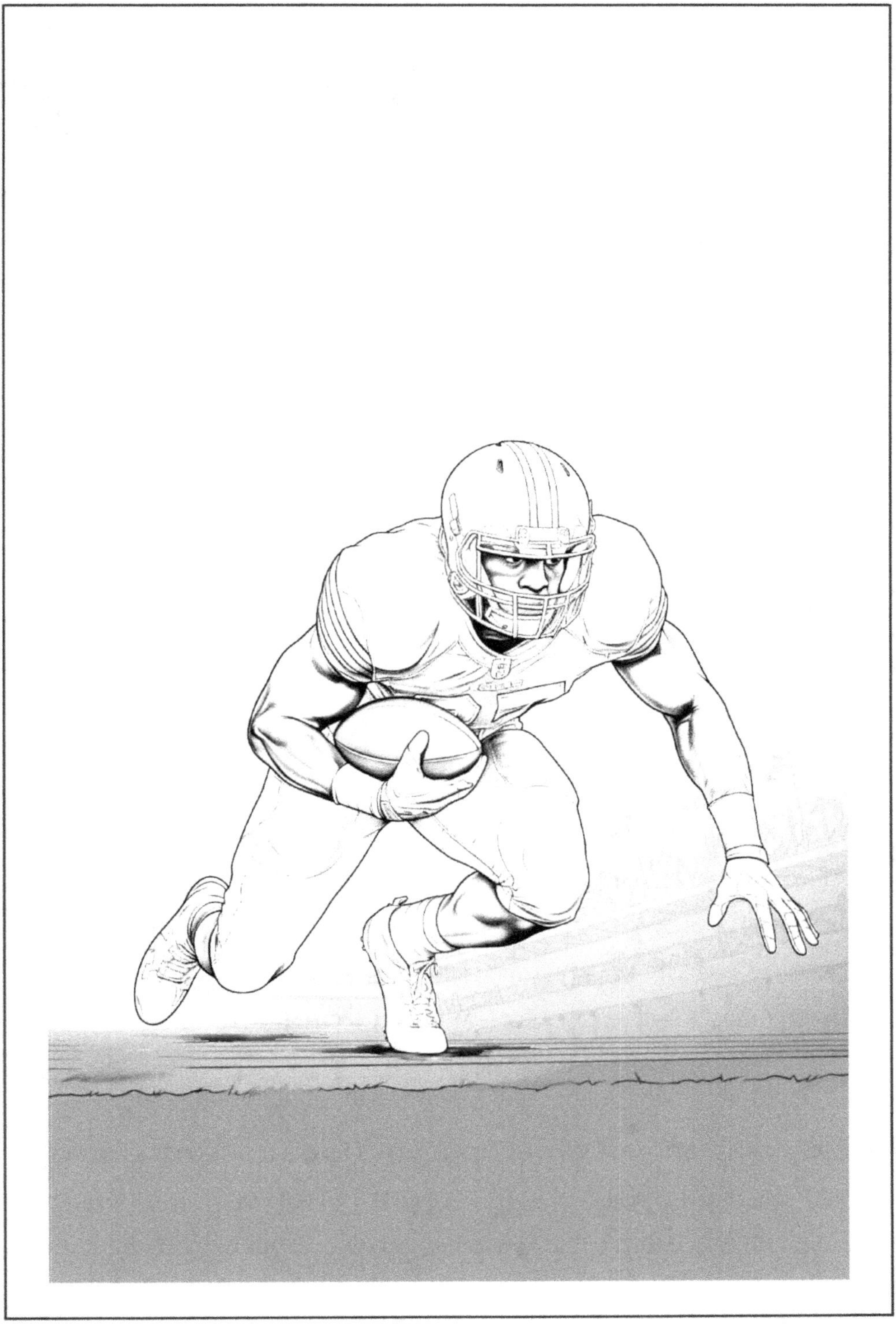

CHAPTER 2

THE FUMBLE FIASCO

So there are a few (well, more than a few) fumble fiascoes to choose from throughout American football history. But, here's one that you'll enjoy!

In January 1987, during a division championship game, the Cleveland Browns faced off against the Denver Broncos. With less than five minutes remaining on the clock and the Broncos having recently extended their lead by seven points, the Browns pinned all their hopes on star quarterback Bernie Kosar to engineer a game-changing play. Imagine being Kosar—the pressure was well and truly on!

Early in the game, Denver appeared to be coasting toward yet another Super Bowl. It began when Elway threw a TD pass to one of the wide receivers, and in a short but suspenseful sequence of events, the Broncos continued to score. Poor Cleveland were only able to score a field goal and the Broncos led 28-3 at halftime.

Things turned around in the third quarter. Kosar threw a few TDs, and running back Earnest Byner scored twice. And by the time the fourth quarter rolled around, Kosar managed to find Webster Slaughter to tie the game.

Scanning the field with unwavering determination, Kosar focused in on the end goal and tried again—he had hope, it looked like the upcoming play held promise. He had the reliable running back Earnest Byner. Determined and ready, Kosar took the snap, and he swiftly handed the ball off to Byner.

Byner, a standout performer during the game, caught the pass, and off he sprinted, with agility and speed, he was heading closer and closer to the end zone. Can you imagine how the crowd watched in breathless anticipation as Byner drew nearer to the goal line? Everyone watching was on the edge of their seats.

However, in a heart-wrenching twist of fate, tragedy struck. In a matter of moments, everything changed for the Cleveland Browns. As Byner reached for the end zone, the football slipped from his grasp, falling to the ground. The once-promising play disintegrated before the eyes of the players, fans, and coaches—the whole stadium was in shock. What a way for things to go; it was a mockery. It makes you think about how things don't always turn out as you hoped. But the game has to go on, and there is no time to feel bad for Byner. Elway and the Broncos took over and a few plays and eventually opted to take an intentional safety to drain precious time on the clock.

Down by five points, they managed to stop the Browns on a Hail Mary attempt, and the game ended in a 38-33 Broncos win. Cleveland went home, but it wasn't all roses for Denver because they then went on to lose to the Washington Redskins in Super Bowl XXII. It is a chapter in football history observed by the erratic hand of fate, with its blend of heartbreak and the unpredictability of the game.

That sinking feeling when you make a mistake—like forgetting to take out the trash or letting the dog out when you weren't supposed to—feels horrible, doesn't it?. Yes, there are consequences, maybe you may lose privileges for a bit or get told off, but it's important to remember that mistakes happen—none of us are perfect, not even top NFL stars. The trick is that you grow and learn from those mistakes so they don't happen again, and remember that you can't be too hard on yourself.

Why? You won't learn much from being too hard (or negative) on yourself. What should you do instead? Stop, think, and then ask why it happened and what changes you can make. What can you remember to help you the next time? How can you stop yourself from repeating the mistake in the future? Reflection is a key way to learn how you can improve next time. When you try this, you'll be surprised to find that you can find helpful ways to crush any setbacks that you may face because of your mistakes.

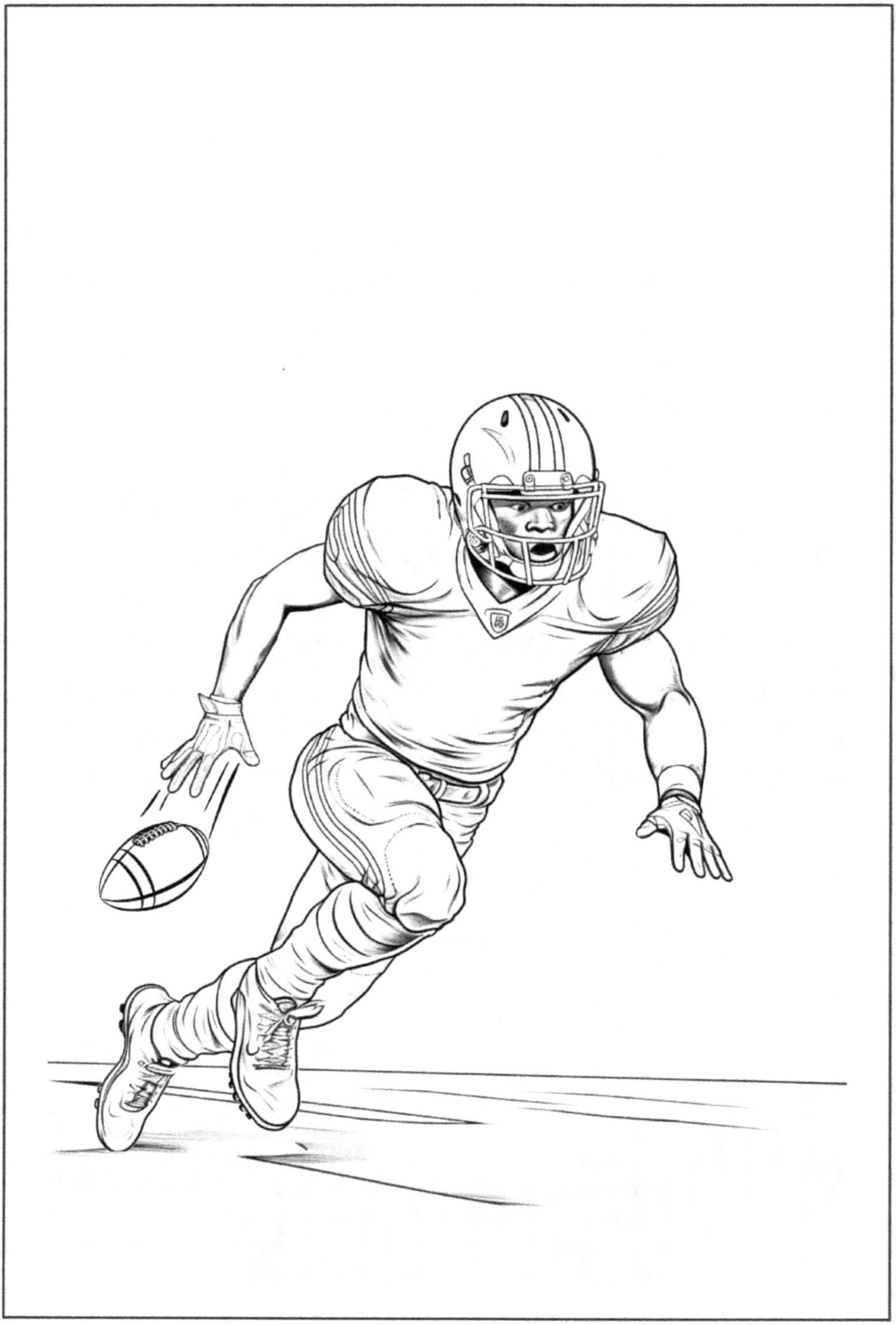

CHAPTER 3

THE ROOKIE SENSATION

Right now, it's the rookie sensation, where a player is in their first ever season of an NFL league game. That has a lot of die-hard fans very excited about the future, but is the risk worth the potential pay-off? If your favorite team signs the right rookie, that could mean great things—at least a playoff run or more. Imagine having to start over again as the New England Patriots who are taking a daring chance on rookie Mac Jones!

With a roaring few seasons under his belt, Jones is defining a new Patriots' era, battling impossible odds and immense expectations. Jones is thriving and inspires confidence in the fans who have a long-storied history with tremendous victory or devastating bust. Will Jones' promising future lead to more Super Bowl wins? Here's to hoping, as Jones tackles an immense responsibility, and works on perfecting his role as the new leader of the Patriots organization. Gosh, many would buckle under the pressure of playing under the shadow of the legendary Tom Brady and working with the mega-coach Bill Belichick.

Most rookie quarterbacks are drafted to teams that don't have winning records with little to no chance of reaching the playoffs - it's too risky. Historically, rookie quarterbacks don't start, let alone win, Super Bowls. Over the last 70 years, only 14 rookies (not counting QBs who stepped in because of injuries) have led their teams to the playoffs in their first appearance—it's a rare occurrence.

As of 2022, Jones joined the ranks of rookie quarterbacks with winning records. His impressive milestones include becoming the 15th rookie quarterback in the league's history to pass for over 3,000 yards and tossing 20 touchdowns.

That's it! No more numbers because I'll have you know Jones isn't just about the numbers; he's earned the respect and admiration of his teammates. And do you know who else is singing Jones's praises? His coach, Bill Belichick. Nothing but praise (in Belichick's classic, no-nonsense way, that is) for Jones's character, focus, and dedication to refining his skill. It will be exciting to see what kind of team the Patriots will become during the Mac Jones era.

We all know how important it is to listen to instructions, no matter how hard, especially when trying to impress your new teammates, coaches, and fans. But what if you've never enjoyed the magic of seeing your breath float away on a cold, crisp winter day?

No one would blame you for getting a little lost in that moment. Luckily you're not Jones, one year into playing for the New England Patriots, who went viral in January 2022 for doing just that.

Sure, you have your doubts; it sounds impossible—and downright hilarious.

But it's true. Poor Jones, from humid subtropical Florida, is playing in near-freezing temperatures. Layered up in his warmest winter clothes, Jones is watching his team losing to the Buffalo Bills. Sure, maybe he should have been focused on listening to the instructions from his offensive coordinator, Josh McDaniels. But how could he?

You know those really cold winter days where you can see your own breath in the air? This, known as a condensation trail, absolutely fascinated Jones on that meme-worthy January day. After watching the first "breath trail," Jones quickly followed up with a few more quick puffs—a viral moment that made most fans laugh! During all this, what did he forget to do? That's right—he forgot to listen to his coordinator.

Let's face it — we've all been there. Blowing trails of cold breath is fascinating, but not as important as listening to instructions.

Listening to instructions is a necessary life skill; imagine you're about to start a project. At first, your teacher will give you instructions, what they expect, and the due date. Initially, these instructions might seem like information overload, or you may be tempted to figure out shortcuts so that the project can be easier or take less time to complete, but what if all that time you spent thinking stopped you from actively listening?

Active listening usually sets you up for success—it will help you understand your goals, what tools you need to complete the project, and how to get the best grade possible. With all of this information, planning and giving yourself enough time to produce an imaginative and creative project will be easier. By having a well-thought-out plan of action, you give yourself a chance to be successful and I'll bet your teacher will be impressed by how responsible you were and that you were taking the project seriously. Don't forget that your teachers are there to help you succeed, so make sure you are always listening—it pays off.

Listening to instructions is a skill that helps you to improve on what you already know, and it also pushes you to be a better person with a stronger character—you may find yourself willing and able to tackle new challenges, lead by a positive example, or be a better friend. Enjoy the fun little moments in life, but don't let them distract you from what's important. So, I hope you're ready to be a better listener and open the doors to exciting opportunities.

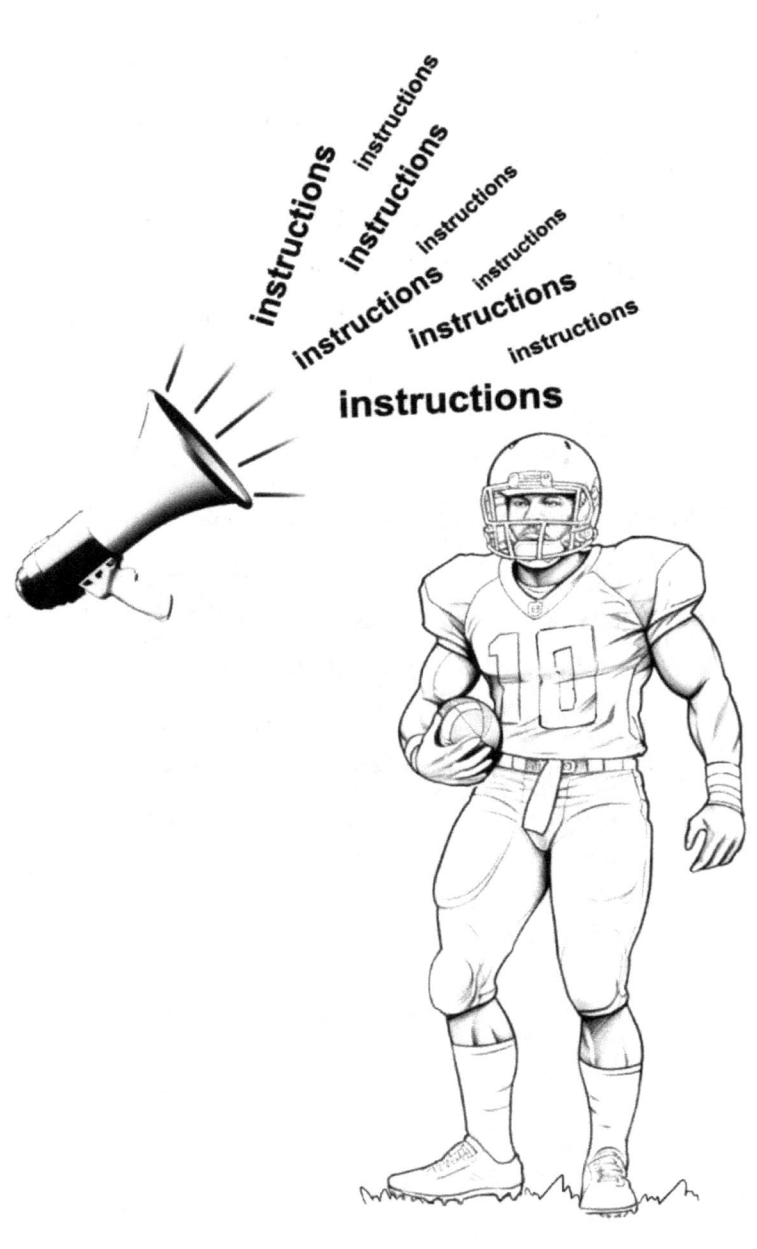

CHAPTER 4

THE TOUCHDOWN CELEBRATION EXTRAVAGANZA

Celebrating your achievements is cool and well-deserved when you work hard to achieve them. How you celebrate is all that matters afterwards, whether it's a gold star, extra recess, or a pizza party! American football players are no different to you and me, especially when celebrating a touchdown. While celebrating a TD isn't new, no one has made it as popular as former Cincinnati Bengals wide receiver Chad Johnson. Also known as Chad Ochocinco, he was never afraid to celebrate his touchdown drives.

Some famous and hilarious celebrations include the following:

Chad caught a 36-yard pass during the second quarter to put the Bengals in the lead. Once he returned to the sidelines, he celebrated the TD by putting on a poncho and sombrero.

Sometimes, his antics got him into trouble and, sometimes, he had to pay fines. Just in case you missed it though, behind all the loud and funny celebrations, Ochocinco has a real heart of gold. Once, after scoring a TD, he grabbed a sack and started handing out autographed footballs like he was Santa Claus—imagine being a fan in the stands receiving an autographed football from Ochocinco. Ho ho ho—Christmas came early!

All that Christmas magic didn't help the Bengals win that game, unfortunately.

Another popular Ochocinco TD dance was his funny version of a jig known as the Riverdance. (The Riverdance was a theater play and a dance honoring Irish culture.) When Chad discovered the traditional Irish dance, he was inspired to do his version to add a bit of a cultural flair that he didn't think happened often enough in American football. And his fancy footwork helped Ochocinco land a spot on a popular television show called Dancing With the Stars, but we won't get into that.

Did you know one time Chad jokingly performed CPR to revive a ball after a TD? It's a shame that the gift of life for the ball didn't help the Bengals win against the Jacksonville Jaguars.

Celebration time can be done in many ways; it doesn't have to be big. Sometimes, it's okay to celebrate on your own—believing and expressing your happiness in a way that feels right for you is the most important thing. Do a little happy dance, treat yourself to your favorite dessert, or wear your best outfit. If your zone is the great outdoors, consider planning an adventure—you can go on a walk, rollerblade, skateboard, play basketball, bike ride, or spend a relaxing day at the splash pad.

Take a moment to be creative. Sometimes, adding your personality and imagination makes your victories more memorable and unique. Why are Ochocinco's TD celebrations remembered? That's right! He had fun, went out of his way, and dared to be different! Enjoying your successes is important, but you should know that you don't boast. Victories are precious, so celebrating is as much about being positive as building self-confidence!

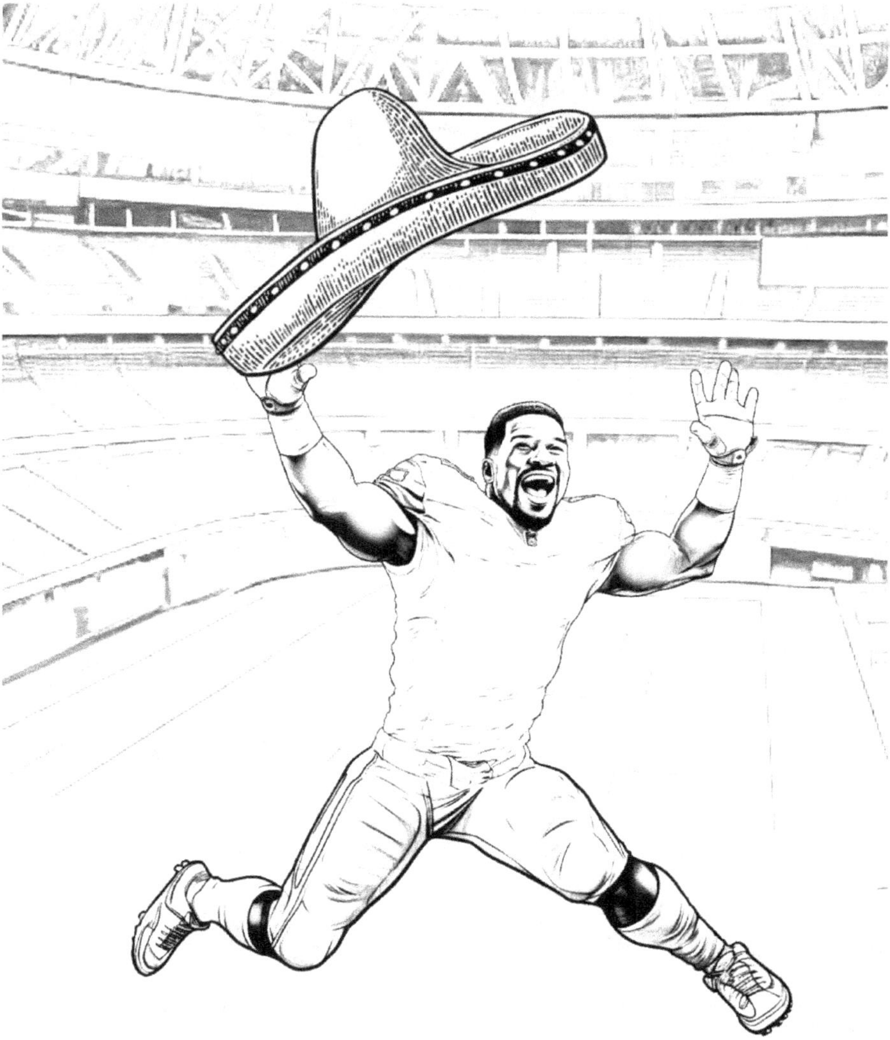

CHAPTER 5

WHEN YOU WISH

One special event happens every year around Christmas. Johnson's organization takes kids on a merry shopping spree—whatever they can grab in 80 seconds is theirs to keep. How exciting is that? Would you believe that the Texans' organization kept this amazing thing a secret for a long time? Supposedly, during one trip, he spent almost $20,000.

Why did he do it? It was because he spent his career focused on giving back to the community and it was a chance for kids who rarely celebrate the little things that other kids may take for granted. And why? Just to give them a chance to enjoy some really fun moments. Are there some things in life you take for granted that others may not have?

Anyway, let's talk about a genuine hero, Andre Johnson (wide receiver for primarily the Houston Texans), who uses his celebrity status to award wishes, which isn't surprising because Johnson was committed to charity and giving back during his career.

He spent most of his career playing for the Houston Texans' and his heroic efforts helped carry this rookie team to great places in its early years. He was one of their best players, leading on and off the field. Like many of you, he fell in love with the game when he was around six or seven years old, and by the time he was in high school, his family and friends started helping him to do whatever they could to help him take care of his gift, whether it was playing multiple sports or traveling 30 miles to attend Miami Senior High School.

Johnson excelled and played for the Hurricanes, the University of Miami football team.

Did you know he caught a 32-yard pass in his first game and scored his first TD? How incredible is that!? And he carried his winning ways into the bigs when he pushed his team in an exciting victory against the Miami Dolphins, gaining around 80 yards. He did such a great job during his rookie season that he was selected for the All-Rookie Team.

As a rookie in 2003, Johnson also created an organization, the Andre Johnson Foundation, to help young kids raised by single parents—the organization hosts events, teaches and supports kids in academics, and helps create positive life skills.

While less funny than most of the stories that are packed here, I couldn't pass up the opportunity to highlight an important lesson: The smallest act can make all the difference.

So what can you do to make your mark? Maybe start off with asking your parents or your school to help you and your friends organize and host an American football-themed bake sale or clothing drive in your community or at your school. Raise some money for a local charity!

You can volunteer at local shelters or food banks; some ways to help include serving or preparing meals, sorting donated items, or taking part in clothing drives. This is a great work experience option if you're a little older. A hands-on experience teaches them the importance of giving to those in need and is a real-world demonstration that small acts of kindness and generosity can make.

Maybe you're not good with talking to people or want to take part in an activity that allows you to listen to nature or your music—consider taking part in clean-up events at local parks or beaches; a great way to do your part and get in touch with nature as you protect it.

And since creativity doesn't have any age limits, consider having an art or talent show for a chance to sell your arts and crafts at local markets (or perform at your local library or community center)—there are so many fun ideas you and your friends can try. Talk to your art teacher to get some inspiration!

So, in your action plan, try setting personal goals to perform acts of kindness each month or school year. Start small, maybe help your siblings with their homework, and help your parents bring in the groceries before being asked; these small acts make a big difference.

Being involved shows compassion and is a fantastic way to show and understand the importance of giving back.

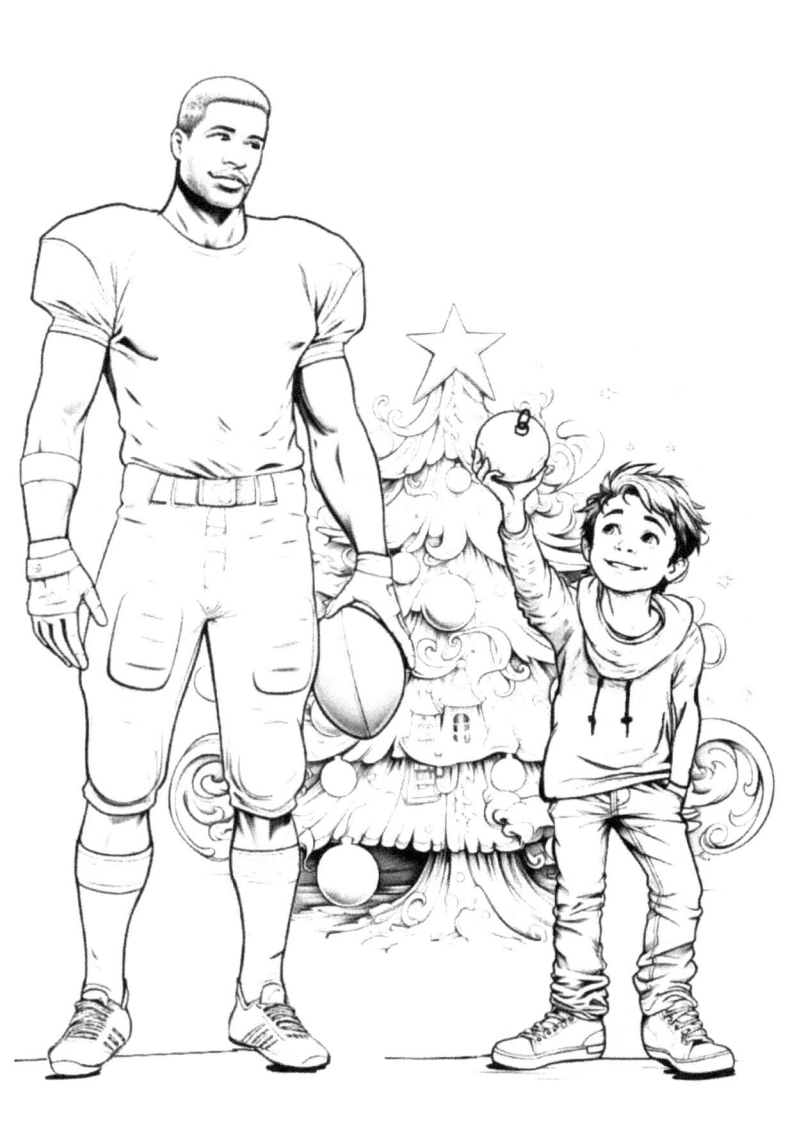

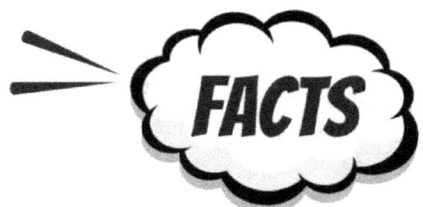

1. American football originated from soccer and rugby.

2. Football began in 1869.

3. American football is called gridiron because it's played on a grassy field like rugby. Since the late 19th century, the sport has been called "gridiron," from the Irish word "gadir," meaning "grid" or "gridiron."

4. The most popular sport in America is football.

5. The Gallaudet University deaf huddle was established in 1894 to hide their sign language from other teams.

CHAPTER 6

THE LEGENDARY QUARTERBACK

After a quarterback gets drafted, the team sets him up for upcoming success. Some teams offer a slower, easy-does-it approach, allowing their quarterbacks to build themselves up, like when you first play a game like Minecraft. You're stuck running around, scared of the Nether. Or when you play a challenge, and there are so many people everywhere, and you run into that player that keeps defeating you, and now you're spectating, waiting for the round to end, so that you can try again.

What makes a quarterback legendary? Is it being on the right team? Is it having the best teammates? Or, is it the coaches and training staff?

Time's up!

So, what did you come up with? Did your answers include being drafted higher or lower in the draft? Was it having your family to support you? Or siblings to challenge you?

I am thinking of legends like the Manning brothers, Eli and Payton, Jim Kelly, Dan Marino, or Andrew Luck. These men have done a lot to change the game. In 2021, five quarterbacks were drafted in the first round, and we talked about one of them back in Chapter Three (Mac Jones).

Let's start by finding a quarterback with the most yards, wins, most championship rings, or maybe a fan favorite that never won a championship.

Even the legends have bad times so it's important to know you can still make an impression and to remember you can make your own luck if you are humble, learn from your mistakes, and will work hard.

Check out this draft report:

- Draft pick, number 199 in the sixth round.

- Pocket-style passer.

- Height advantage, ability to have a superb view across the field.

- Alert and composed.

It sounds like a player that may have lasted for a season or two and probably the last person you'd pick for a game of tag. Well, just so you know, it's the report of the former quarterback of the New England Patriots, Tom Brady—an American Football legend.

Shocking! It seemed everyone figured Brady would be a student with Cs and Ds, but he was an A++ student of the game when you look at that report again.

The Unforgettable Comeback in 2017—time is ticking down, less than 20 minutes to go in Super Bowl LI, the New England Patriots were on their way to losing to the Atlanta Falcons. With the third quarter almost over, how did Tom Brady solve the puzzle, push his team to an incredible comeback, and win their fifth title in overtime? Well, scoring 25 unanswered points to tie the game added to the momentum, and Patriots running back James White's extension into the end zone was also an enormous help. Also, Brady's emotional reason for digging deep and giving it his best shot showcases his unbreakable spirit.

Anyway, after all that drama, would you believe the Patriots pushed through their obstacles and won the championship with a touchdown on the first drive of overtime? Tom Brady's journey is a story of wins, losses, gaining weight (physically and mentally, aka willing to learn), and the will to rise above challenges to prove himself. From being an underdog draft pick to directing stunning comebacks, not letting his age define him, and having the courage to start again with a new team, Tom's story teaches us that even the most outstanding people face challenges, just like you and me.

So, what valuable lessons can we take from Tom Brady's journey? We should welcome challenges with open arms, strive for excellence and never give up. Tom Brady's story shows that when you believe in yourself and dream big, who knows what great things you can accomplish?

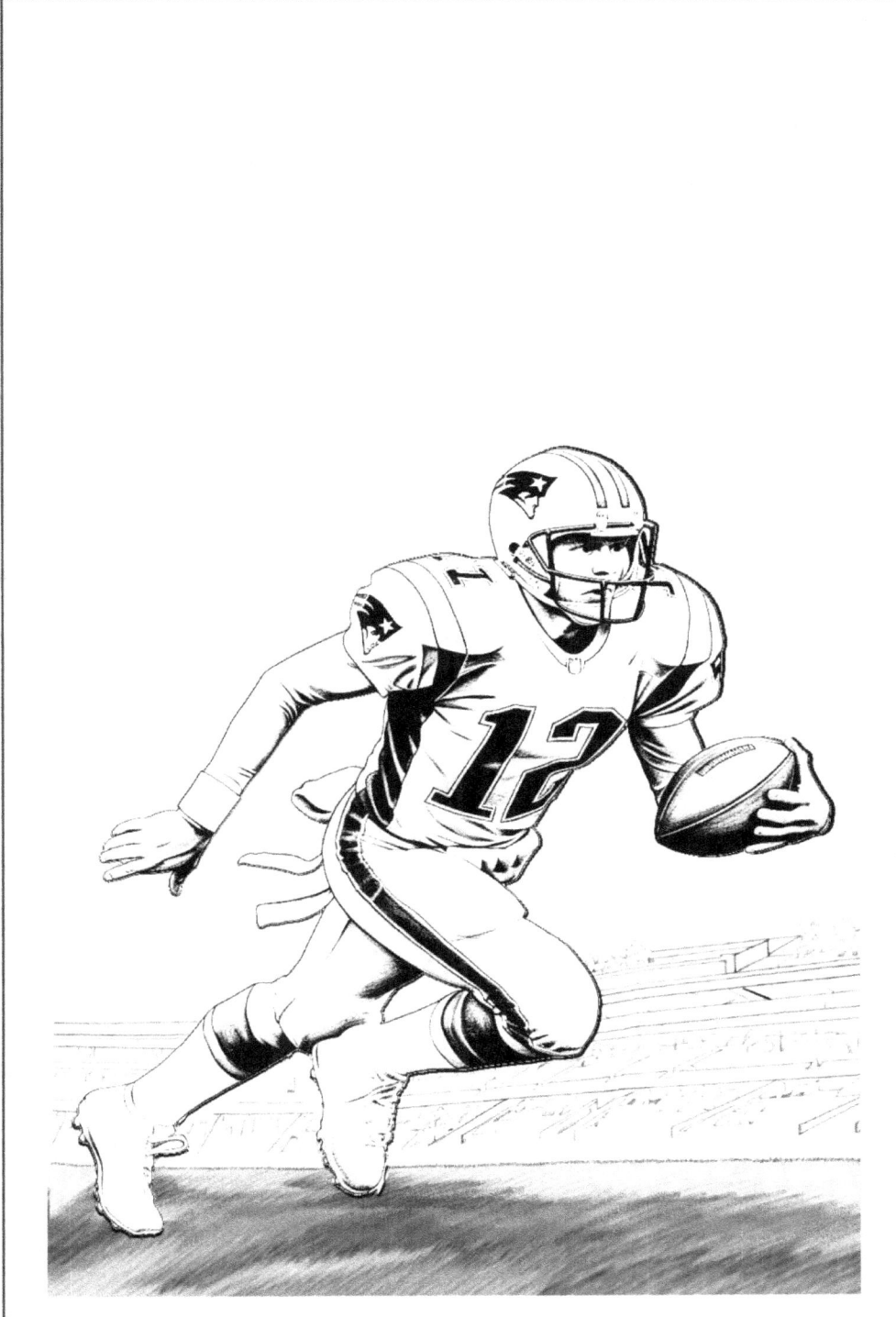

CHAPTER 7

THE FOOTBALL MAGICIAN

Sometimes magic on the field comes from your inner strength, no, no, not your physical strength—the magic inside you. Here is the story of former long punter Jon Dorenbos. At 12 years old, Jon moved to a new neighborhood. Soon after moving in, Jon was introduced to a teenage magician and found hope; magic became the way for Jon to find "a really cool place." (He practiced a lot and, in eighth grade, he won a talent show at school!)

As Jon grew older, one of his classmates a few years later suggested he should try out for American football. Jon was a big, sturdy kid, but he decided that he would still prefer to work on his magician skills. But his classmate insisted, pointing out that magic and the game of football are similar and explained how the right plays can change the course of the game to push your team to victory. What magician doesn't like a sleight of hand or conjuring their best at will?

When Jon started high school, he joined the football team and played at the long snapper position, excelling at 15-yard precision hikes or snaps. Playing football made Jon feel strong and part of a big team. He worked really hard and got impressively good at the sport. Now, Jon was not only a fantastic magician but a skilled football player too! His magic tricks were as remarkable as his hikes and his punts and eventually he gravitated toward the long snapper position.

What is a long snapper?

No, it has nothing to do with fishing or the sound you make with your fingers.

A long snapper's job is like the center, the player responsible for hiking or snapping the ball to the quarterback. Long snappers are on the field when their team is looking to score a field goal or make an attempt for extra points. It's certainly an important job with a lot of responsibility.

Jon created a VHS package (like a story or a highlight reel). He sent it to various colleges—the package may have included a few creative adjustments (think filters or hashtags) to highlight Jon's skills. Jon won a college scholarship to the University of Texas at El Paso (UTEP), became a top long snapping prospect, and spent over a decade playing football.

In 2016, while Jon was playing for the Philadelphia Eagles, Jon auditioned for the TV show America's Got Talent (AGT).

Why is "laces out" a magical play?

It's alllllll-punt-righty!

Horrible pun-t attempt.

Anyway, Jon took a chance and bet on himself. He had nothing to lose, and why not? He had to try, and I'll bet he assumed he would be eliminated from the show before training camp was over.

And, we know magic doesn't work like that, right?

Anyway, Jon decided not to tell the Eagles because he didn't think the team would find out about it, but guess what? The team owners found out about the appearance and thought it was super neat. And, just like that, for just a moment, Jon's life became a terrific combination of football, magic, and joy. Sadly, he didn't win the competition, but he had a fantastic time.

So, you see, Jon Dorenbos showed us that even when life is tough, if you believe and embrace your magic and do everything with purpose and passion, you can be outstanding at more than one thing. Jon's story reminds us that hard work can make our dreams come true, and a few spells never hurt.

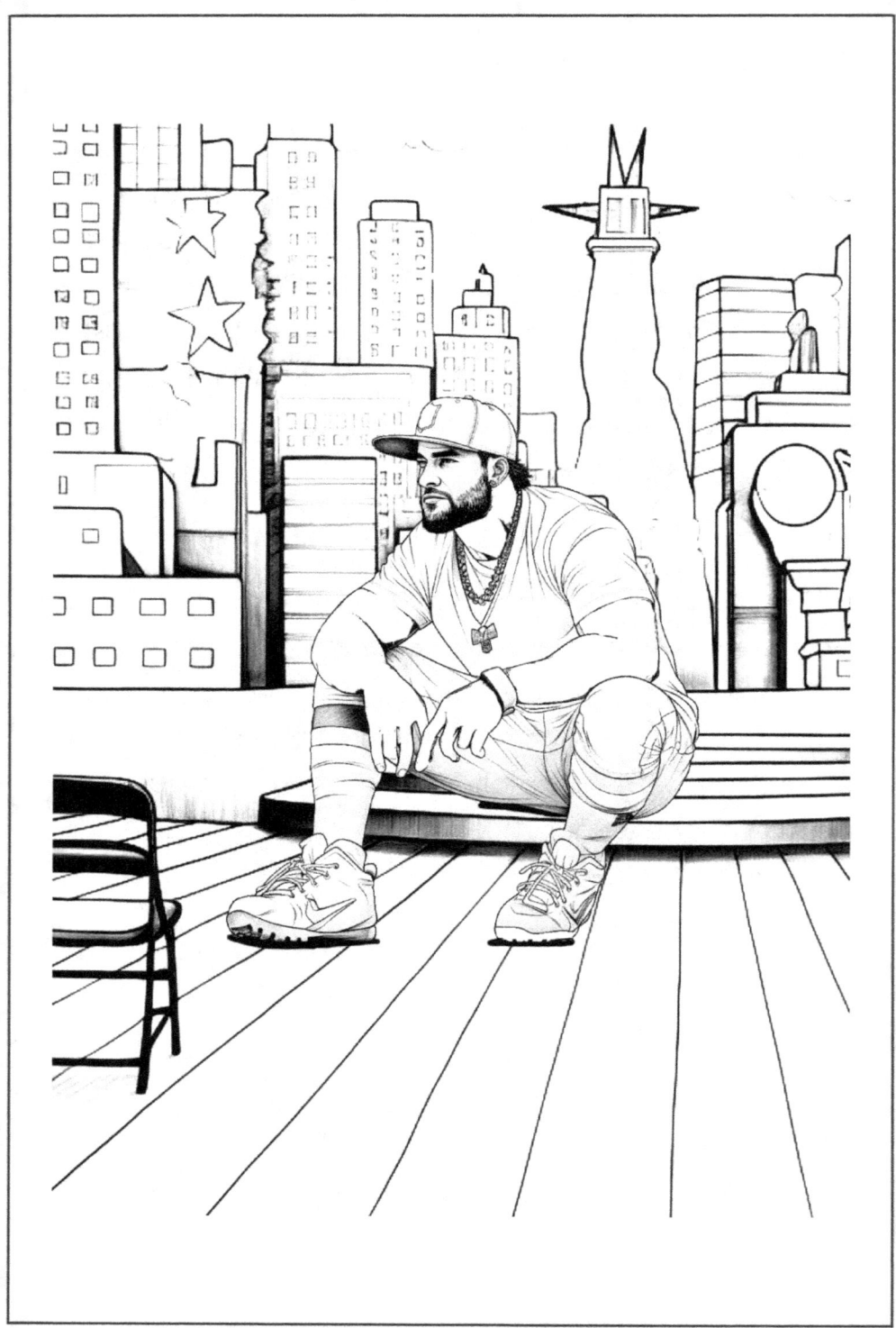

CHAPTER 8

THE BEAUTY OF BEAST MODE

OMarshawn Lynch grew up in Oakland, California, and he dreamed of playing football when he was younger. He played football at the University of California before the Buffalo Bills signed him in the 2007 draft. A few years later, Marshawn was signed by the Seattle Seahawks, where he began shining even brighter. His genuine affection and respect for his new team were hard to contain and, eventually, his hard work led to his first championship win during Super Bowl XLVIII.

On the field, Marshawn's deceptive running style always made magic, and his dazzling displays, whether juking or confusing defenders, allowed Marshawn to run over them. His style is distinctive in American football and back in the 2010-2011 playoff season, Marshawn destroyed his competitors with various power moves with unique names like Beast Quake. Marshawn Lynch is known for his Beast Mode style, which has become his unofficial (official) nickname. With his ability to drive and create plays with the force of his will, players and coaches alike are amazed at Lynch's unique blend of incredible strength and admirable skills.

Lynch had an amazing career, with over 9,000 rushing yards and nearly 75 touchdowns under his belt in his 10-year American football career.

Lynch was a fan-favorite who loved Skittles and was a dominant force at the core of the Seahawks offense. During one game, Lynch ran for over 65 yards and almost had double digits in broken tackles, helping his team win a crucial playoff game against the New Orleans Saints.

In one game back 2018, Lynch, who was now playing for the Raiders', started another season in fine fashion. "Beast Mode" style, of course. So, on the first drive, with the ball around second, and goal, the Raiders quarterback handed the ball off to Marshawn Lynch, who went full "Beast Mode", connecting and dragging the defense yards away out from the end zone—with a bit of wind, sorry a "push" from his offensive line, Lynch would continue pushing and jostling before shoving the pile of players ahead for the score.

While success usually depends on more than individual talent, you need a sprinkle of strength, a dash of humbleness, unwavering dedication, and the power of encouragement. Acting with integrity is necessary. What is integrity? Integrity is treating everyone well, no matter what, with respect and heart. You should always put your best foot forward and encourage your inner Beast Mode to shine. Like Marshawn, you can use humor and a light-hearted approach to life to uplift those around you. Why? Encouraging others and showing kindness can be a positive push to help you show others how they can reach their full potential—the sky is the limit.

Lynch's drive shows success often needs constant work toward reaching your goals. It's a reminder that ambitions and faith are the key. So, what's stopping you from beginning your trip to achieving greatness?

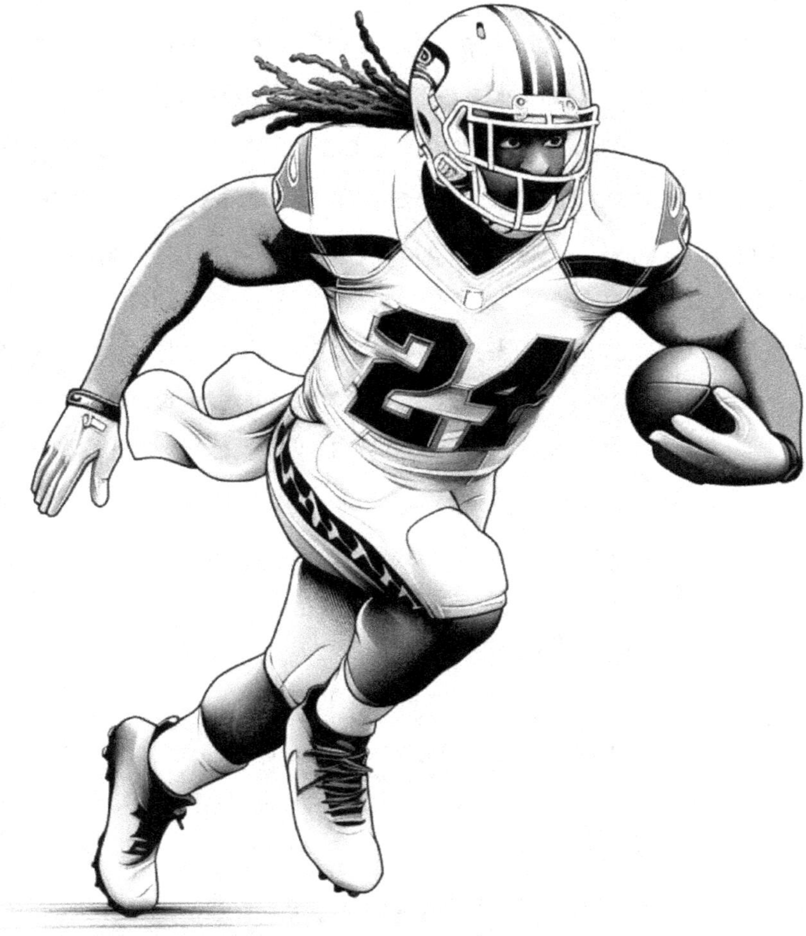

CHAPTER 9

PHILLY, PHILLY—OH, SO SPECIAL!

Imagine playing in the championship game, and a trick play brings your team toward an unlikely destiny. A chance, a moment to win the biggest prize of all!

So, this magical moment happened during Super Bowl LII. The Philadelphia Eagles were facing the New England Patriots, and everyone thought the Patriots had a lock on winning the game. But a clever, creative play just before halftime became an amazing play that will be remembered for a very long time.

The Eagles had a 15-12 lead over the Patriots on the Patriots 1-yard line, less than 40 seconds away from the half. It would've been safe to just go for the field goal, but the Eagles coach opted for the TD. Why not? It doesn't hurt to take a chance, especially when playing against Bill Belichick, Tom Brady, and the rest of the defending Championship (2017) Patriots.

What happened next has been called the Philly, Philly aka The Philly Special. The Eagles coach told his quarterback, Nick Foles, to get ready for a piece of history-making trickery! The coach had Foles line up behind the offensive line, then asked the center (Jason Kelce) to snap the ball to the closest running back, who tossed the ball to the left into the hands of a nearby tight end. The tight end, Corey Burton, took off and began charging toward the end zone. Distraction mode: activated! This left the Patriots focused on the wrong players and missing out on the fact that Foles was open; the ball sailed into his hands, and he scored the touchdown.

The Eagles won the game, and Foles became the first quarterback to throw and catch for a TD in a Champion game. What a game! Their daring ways show that risk-taking can lead to magical success with great pay-off.

So, back to you; what do you think this means? First, you want to take chances, be curious, be proud of the things you're good at, and enjoy the things that make you unique. Next, you can work on your strengths and weaknesses to help you work better with others and yourself. It will help you keep a positive attitude, accept and learn when you deal with constructive criticism, or be brave enough to try new (and unique) ideas—you will also be able to be consistent and dedicated. How? When you are dedicated to a person or an idea, you will keep trying and pushing yourself even when you feel like giving up. There's always a solution, and with dedication you're sure to find it. With practice, you will use what you've learned to be creative and to use them to create your own path to success. Think about what the Eagles did in the Championship; they could've been happy with a smaller lead or being behind, but because they took a chance and went for a TD, it boosted the team's confidence and pushed them to victory. It's time to believe in yourself and be proud of what makes you unique—these are important tools for success.

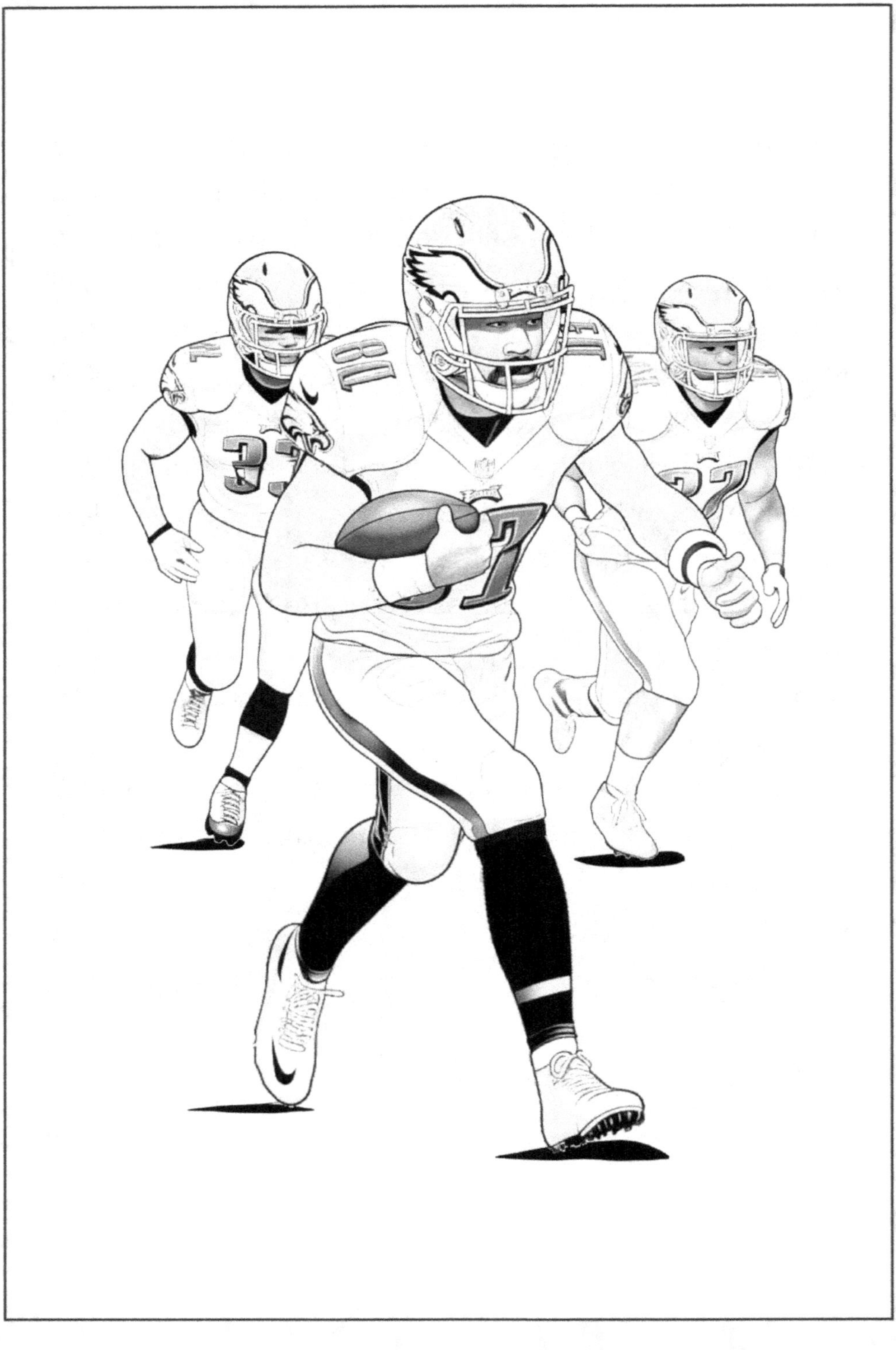

CHAPTER 10

THE COMEBACK KINGS

Do a little dance, emote the Floss, and give it up for the winner of the best comeback to date: the 1993 Buffalo Bills. While many other teams have celebrated glorious comebacks, they are not known as "The Comeback."

This particular comeback, "The Comeback", featured the Bills against the Houston Oilers (now Tennessee Titans) in the first round of a divisional playoff game. They were already down by over 30 points in the third quarter. This was a game that showcased the true essence of resilience and determination. Those poor Bills fans had probably lost all hope—things look pretty bad when your team is losing by that many points. You cling on to any little bit of hope that things may, as they say, make a comeback.

Can you imagine how many of their fans had already given up and were counting down the minutes to what seemed like an inescapable defeat, preparing themselves for great disappointment? How many fans believed the Bills could come back, searching for that so-called hope? Watching the Oilers' dominant performance had left little room for any optimism for the Bills fans in the stadium, and those watching from home. Also, it didn't help that the Bills star quarterback, Jim Kelly, suffered a right knee sprain during the last game of the regular season. This left the Bills no other option but to rely on the backup, Frank Reich—the odds really weren't in their favor that day.

Now, back to that game. So, before the second half began, Bills coach Marv Levy gave a rallying speech and he reminded the players that they had to dig deep to make a comeback. Guess what? It worked, Marv had tapped into a wavelength that motivated and appealed to the players' emotions and pride.

What happened next was an unforgettable and legendary performance by the team and their backup quarterback. Reich transformed and led the Bills on an incredible journey of redemption; the Bills launched a scoring spree that would exceed expectations. Precision pass after precision pass, Reich stepping up and leading his team. Completion after completion, the momentum started shifting, and the points were mounting for the Bills. The previously quiet crowd at Rich Stadium (now Highmark Stadium) hollered and roared. Each touchdown and successful play sparked magic in that stadium. The Oilers struggled to contain their fragile hold on the lead but couldn't hold on. The game was tied at 38-38. While each team fought with everything they had to stay in the playoffs, Buffalo's 41-38 victory was eventually sealed by a successful field goal, making it the largest comeback in American football history—now that's an accomplishment!

The Comeback reminds us of the power of the human spirit and how important it is to understand that roadblocks aren't the end of our journey—there is always an alternative route. It should be considered a chance to grow, believe, and strive toward being present, especially when our set goals unravel. If we can turn our doubts into faith, both in ourselves and the possibility of a brighter future, it is a powerful force that teaches us setbacks, failures, and hardships are not endpoints but stepping stones on the journey to success. They provide us with the option to reexamine our goals, to adapt, and to be stronger than ever. Remember that decisiveness (taking action) can lead to remarkable achievements in challenging times.

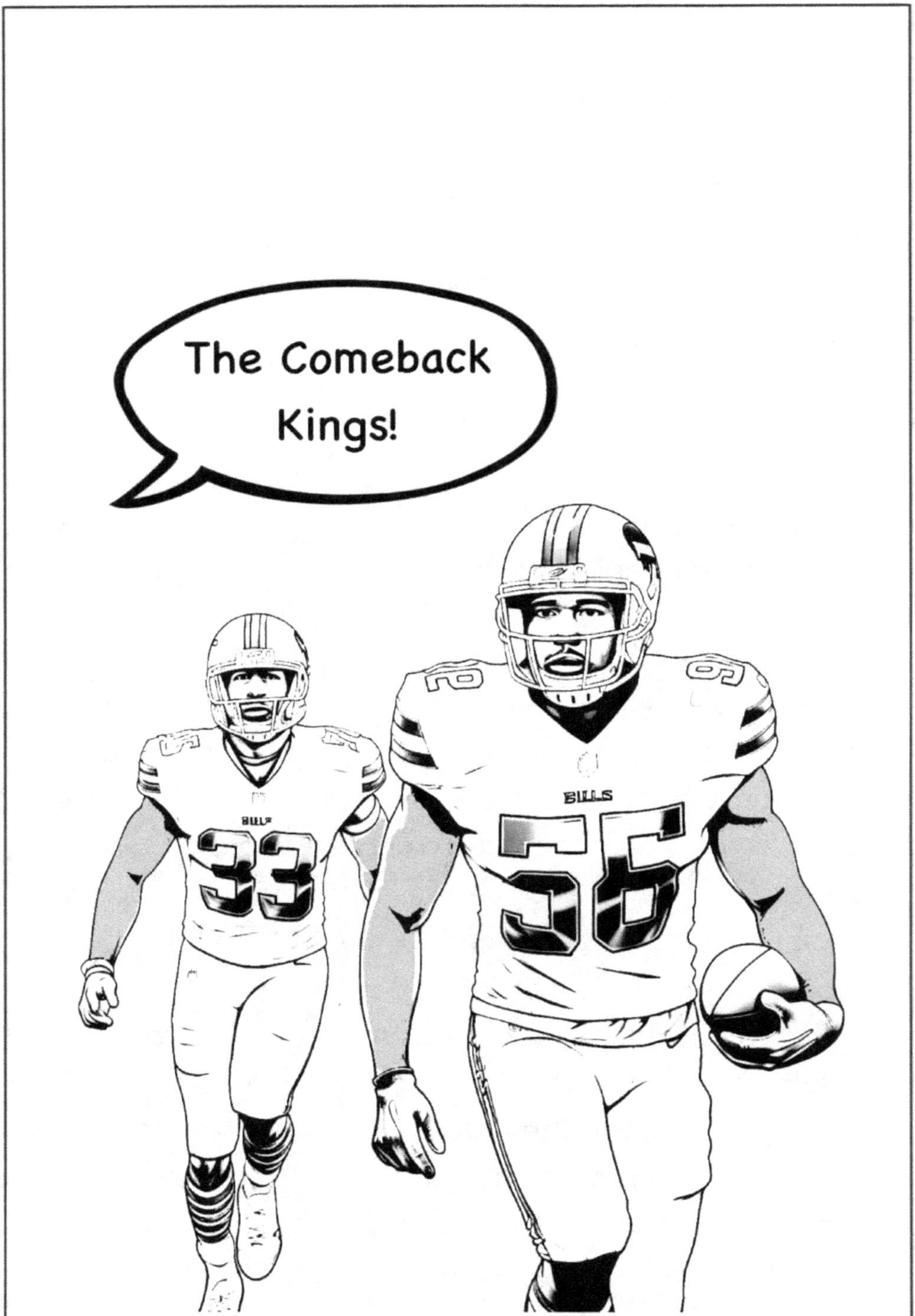

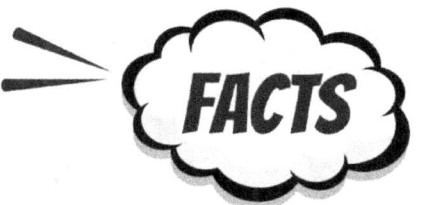

FACTS

1. The Super Bowl is the second-biggest U.S. food day behind Thanksgiving.

2. The NFL's longest field goal is 64 yards.

3. Tiffany & Co. makes the $50,000 Lombardi Trophy for Super Bowl winners.

4. The NFL averages 540,000 footballs every season.

5. The Giants drenched Bill Parcells with Gatorade after a win in 1984, starting the "Gatorade Shower."

CHAPTER 11

THE MVP SIBLINGS

The Kelce brothers (Jason and Travis) share a rare feat in the 2022 season.

See if you can follow me here, it's a little confusing—the Kelce's are not the first pair of brothers to play in the finals and they're not even the first brothers to face each other. BUT they are the first brothers to play on opposite teams at the Super Bowl.

Did you know that Super Bowl LVII was jokingly called the Kelce Bowl, poking a little fun at this rare occasion? It was a temporary way to honor a once-in-a-lifetime event; two brothers playing for opposing teams during the Super Bowl. They were facing each other along with their respective teams: the Kansas City Chiefs (Travis) and the Philadelphia Eagles (Jason).

Imagine being their parents. Who would they root for? On one hand, you have younger brother Travis playing for the Chiefs. On the other, older brother Jason is playing for the Eagles. How do you divide your attention equally? The choice was simple for their mom, Donna—she cheered for both sons. She was even invited to start the game by doing the coin toss, and being the exceptional mom she is, she wore a super multicolored jacket, split down the middle with one side Chiefs and the other half Eagles! She complemented her outfit with a Mama Kelce handbag. On her feet, she decided against donning magical heels of ruby or silver. Instead, she wore sneakers decorated with her sons' jersey numbers: #65 Eagles and #87 Chiefs. What a way to demonstrate her undivided and unconditional love for her sons.

Game time!

After trailing 14-21 at the half, the Chiefs came up with three big offensive plays and three touchdowns in the third and fourth quarters. With just over five minutes left, the Eagles scored another touchdown, tying the game at 35-35 with a successful two-point conversion. Then the Chiefs kicker sealed the deal by kicking a field goal to win the game 38-35.

For Travis, beating his big brother on football's grandest stage was an emotional experience. For Jason, the loss had him contemplating his future, unsure if he would return for another season. (However, he later announced his decision to continue playing for the Eagles, expressing his gratitude for his long-standing career with the team.)

Although playing against each other brought mixed emotions, the Kelce brothers cherished the journey and the moments they shared throughout the historic season. Their bond as brothers remained unbreakable, even in the face of the ultimate football rivalry. After the game, the brothers stopped to hug each other on the field. Their remarkable journeys to the final game illustrated the importance of competition, strength, the lasting bonds of family, and the power of tireless support, both on and off the field. It's a reminder that faced with enormous challenges and intense rivalry, the Kelce brothers never allowed their pursuit of individual success to strain their relationship. Instead, they celebrated each other's achievements. After all, the relationships we encourage honestly represent our victories in life.

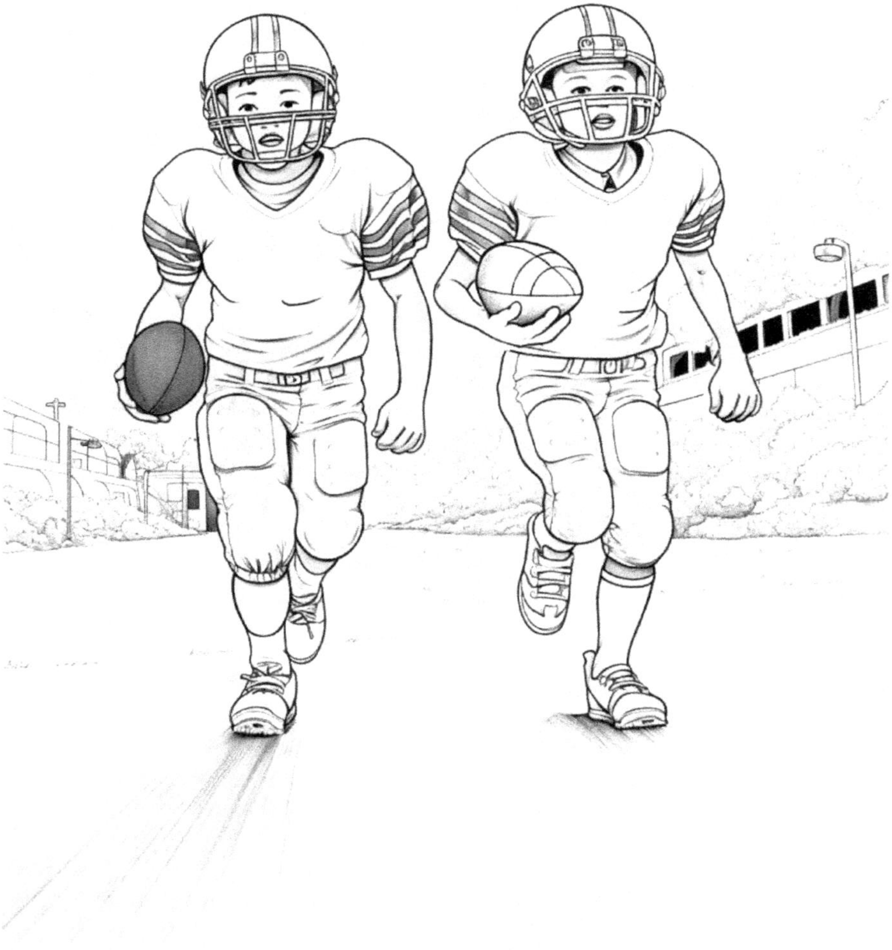

CHAPTER 12

THE SUPER BOWL SURPRISE

The Super Bowl is the marquee event of the year, but sometimes, gosh, the best games are the ones where you are cry-laughing because you could have never guessed what a wild mess these matchups would become. What should be a clear victory turns into a sloppy defeat, the ball develops feelings, the calls aren't benefiting either team, inches turn the tide, or a blowout destroys all hope—it's a beautiful chaos. As it so happens, here is the story of Super Bowl LV when the Tampa Bay Buccaneers beat the Kansas City Chiefs. The Chiefs, led by superstar quarterback Patrick Mahomes, headed into Super Bowl LV as big favorites to defend their Super Bowl crown, especially after dismantling the Buffalo Bulls in the divisional championship game.

So, what was the big plan? The Chiefs' goal was to become the first team to win back-to-back Super Bowls since the

New England Patriots in the early 2000s. And, oh boy, what a huge ambition! However, the quarterback on the opposite touchline to Mahomes was the man who led the Patriots to those consecutive championship victories—Tom Brady. They were aiming to beat that very man's' record. Surprise and awe filled the air as Brady threw three impressive touchdown passes. Then the Bucs' defense went to work and effectively shut down the formerly explosive Kansas offense, limiting the Chiefs to only nine points and no touchdowns.

In sports like hockey, baseball, and soccer, championship games are only played at home or away, and the "home-field advantage" is the idea that when a team plays in their stadium, they have a unique edge because they know the field and have the support of the crowd. There's no place like home—where they feel a deep connection.

Have you figured out the "surprise" yet? By winning Super Bowl LV, the Tampa Bay Buccaneers became the first team in history to win a Super Bowl in their home stadium. It's interesting to note that there's no "home-field advantage" during the Super Bowl because the League reaches out to various cities before the big game and asks the different team owners if they would like to host.

Sometimes, unpredictability and overwhelming circumstances can stop you from even wanting to try. Occasionally, new experiences and situations can make you forget about the things you have accomplished in the past—don't let them overwhelm you, the power is in your hands. Believing in yourself and holding on to your drive with a tight grip to succeed can remind you of the importance of being a leader, using your experience to help you forge alternative paths, and recognizing that you can achieve feats that defy expectations. Sure, life can be unpredictable at times, but don't let the odds and your doubts stop you from reaching new heights and exceeding expectations.

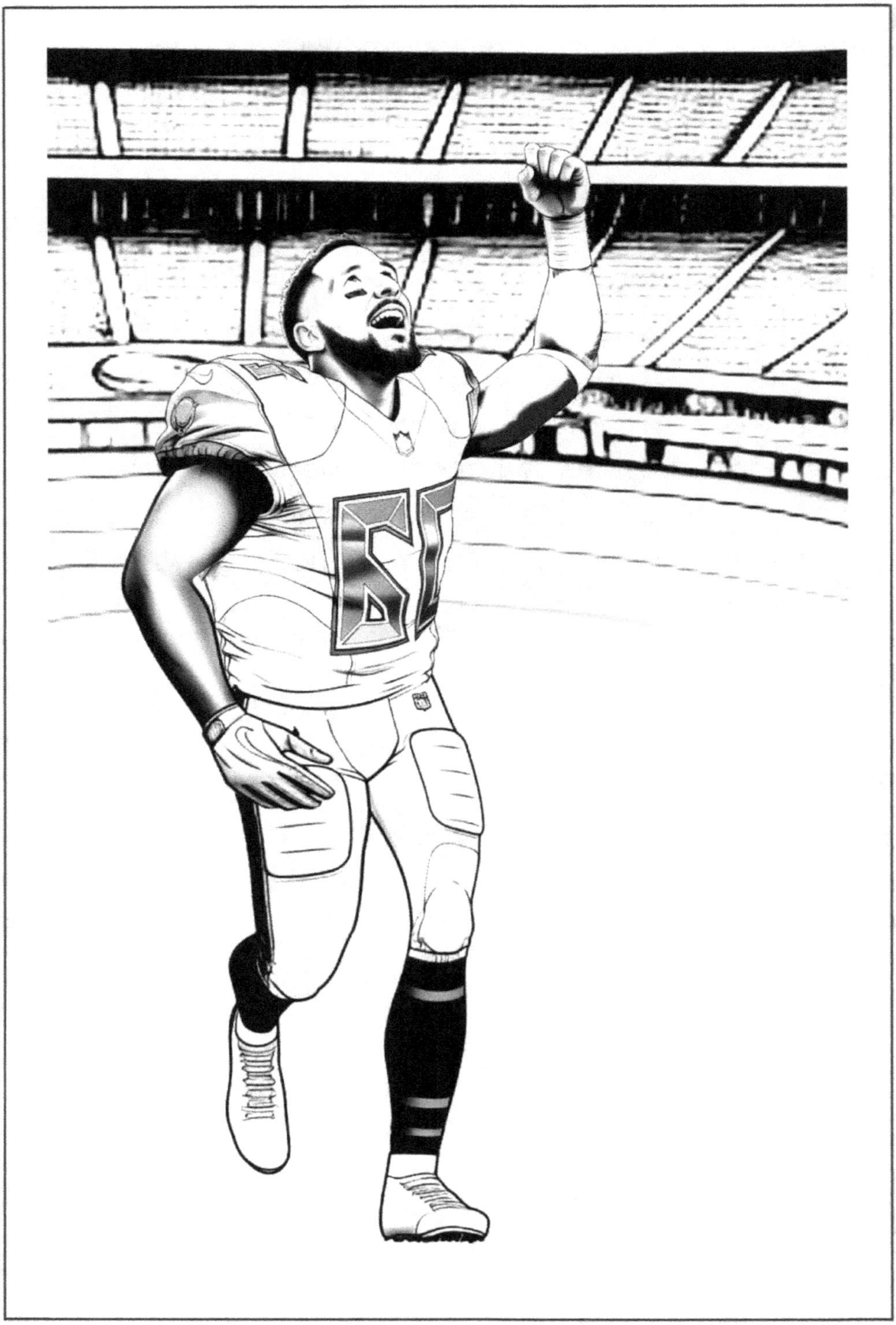

CHAPTER 13

MEGATRON'S MAGICAL HANDS

Few skill-position players were better or more explosive than Calvin Johnson, and his physical traits were almost unparalleled. He became a one-person highlight reel for the Detroit Lions from 2007 through 2015, making it hard to choose which unforgettable moment to discuss. From catches against tough defenders to playing in a snow game or two, those hands caught and completed some stellar touchdowns. With so many extraordinary, talented, determined, and dedicated moments to choose from, which one is the best? It's hard to say, but the moment below is just one story about how legendary and inspiring Calvin Johnson truly was. It is one example of how he earned himself the nickname Megatron.

Back in October 2013, Megatron almost made history for the all-time single-game receiving record against the Dallas

Cowboys in a winning cause. It may never have happened in the explosive way it did if Johnson wasn't inspired by the comments made by Cowboys receiver Dez Bryant. During a radio interview, Bryant said he didn't believe Johnson was the league's best receiver but was looking forward to a fun matchup. Johnson's teammates noticed nothing different, except maybe Johnson seemed more quiet and intense, did he perhaps hear the comments? So, when that Sunday came, no one expected anything but Megatron's regular magic and pregame routine. Before kickoff, he arrived several hours early, walking around the field, visualizing the routes he needed to run, and mentally prepared for the blocks he would need to make. Johnson was making sure he was ready.

Soon, it was game time. Megatron's first catch came early, with less than three minutes left in the first quarter. Little did anyone know this catch would set the fire of a tremendous start.

Feeding off the intense adrenaline of the tens of thousands of cheering fans, Johnson took off on a route—there he goes, running, running, and running. He took a few quick steps before snatching up the ball in the blink of an eye and letting his strength and speed take over and smoothly danced away from an oncoming player near the 25-yard line. Johnson continued outrunning the Dallas defense before the defenders finally caught him and forced him out of bounds for 87 yards on the play. Johnson knew he had the potential to make at least 200 yards that night. As the game continued into the second half, Johnson kept making catch after catch, and no matter how hard the Cowboys tried to slow him down, they failed. He was unstoppable. The Lions won; Megatron was less than 10 yards short of the record set back in 1989 of 15 passes caught for 336 yards. By the way, Johnson finished that afternoon with 14 catches for 329 yards and a touchdown.

What can you do? Let's say you have a talent (even if you don't know what it is yet), it's important to embrace self-motivation to help you accomplish your dreams. Start small, and remember to study extra hard for your test, especially when it's a topic you struggle with. Next, push past your worries and teach yourself to have a little faith in your talents. Even when your friends don't believe in you, you can be your own cheerleader. Be fearless and use those doubts to push you closer to your goals. With clear goals in mind, you'll be surprised at how much easier they are to achieve when you set some goals and start working toward them. Lastly, keep positive people around you. They will help you celebrate your achievements, provide critical (or kind) feedback, and listen to you as you work past obstacles. Bonus points if you help them celebrate their achievements too. So, get to it: How will you overcome challenges and achieve your dreams? Don't let your talents fall behind. Make them a priority and be a witness to all you can achieve.

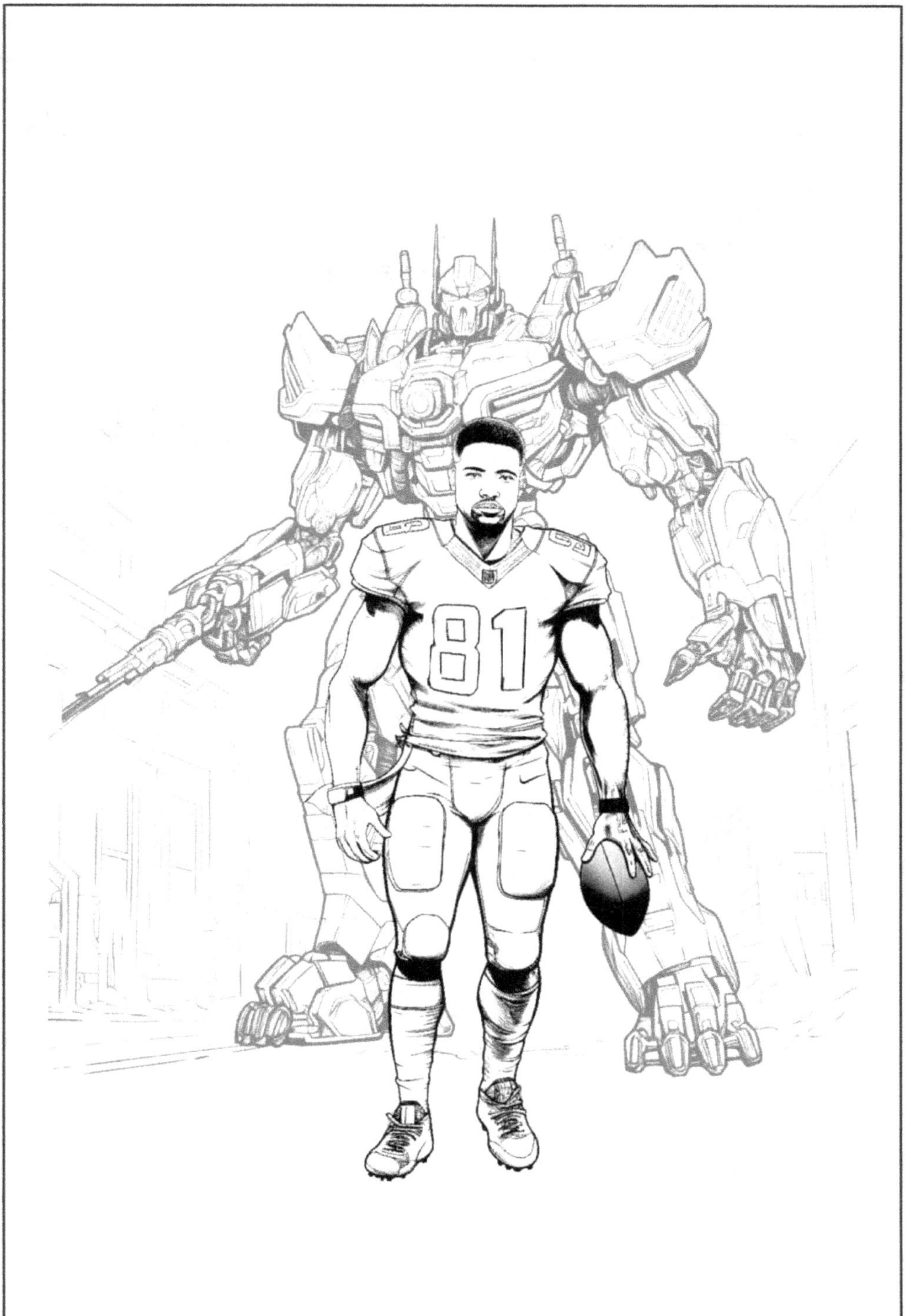

CHAPTER 14

A SWIPE OF THE BRUSH AFTER DASHES AND PASSES: ERNIE BARNES

Playing sports can be an opportunity for a kid who wants to fit in, leave their past behind, and figure out their path. Whether by moving by inches and yards on the field, doodling and making sketches of the sun in the clouds on the sidelines in between plays, or eagerly shouting encouragement to your teammates. Ernie Barnes was a man whose playing days set him up for incredible success as a pioneering artist, an opportunity he wouldn't have had otherwise.

During his playing days, Ernie sometimes got in trouble for drawing during downtime, but that didn't stop him. He was trying to stay calm and focused on the game, and he figured he'd pass the time drawing rather than noticing his breath. If something keeps you relaxed and focused on the upcoming challenges, who's to say you can't be doing it. Ernie would draw linesmen, mimicking their posture and finding creative and often funny ways to capture their movements on the field. When Barnes played in Denver, a sketch he got in trouble for sold for almost ten times the amount he was fined.

He enjoyed five seasons playing professional football, drafted by the Washington Redskins (Commanders). Barnes moved around a lot during his time in the big leagues, also playing for teams like the Baltimore (Indianapolis) Colts, the Titans of New York (NY Jets), and he played his last season for a Canadian team called the Saskatchewan Roughriders. After he retired, the owner of the San Diego Chargers offered Ernie a chance to become the league's official artist—what an opportunity! It helped push Ernie into making his art a viable and exciting career—his art has even been featured on album covers, and his signature style embraces long, lean characters in motion.

What can you learn about yourself when you're brave enough to observe? How can you discover your creativity through problem-solving and never giving up? Like Ernie, you can start by paying close attention to the world around you. Learn to develop keen observation skills so you can be like Ernie, who used his skills to make his art relatable and impactful.

Ernie Barnes's story reminds us that originality and imagination are excellent ways to express ourselves and the things we are passionate about. Sometimes, it might seem the right thing to do, but remember that when we ignore our dreams, wants, and secret talents, we can be our worst enemy. How? By allowing your doubts to get in the way of your chances to grow, you won't learn new things about yourself, and may even miss the opportunity to help and inspire others. Ernie's story reminds us to love what makes us extraordinary and dare to face challenges head-on, even when we think we are already living our best lives. So, let's be bold, and be yourself! What are you passionate about? What steps are you willing to take to make your dreams real?

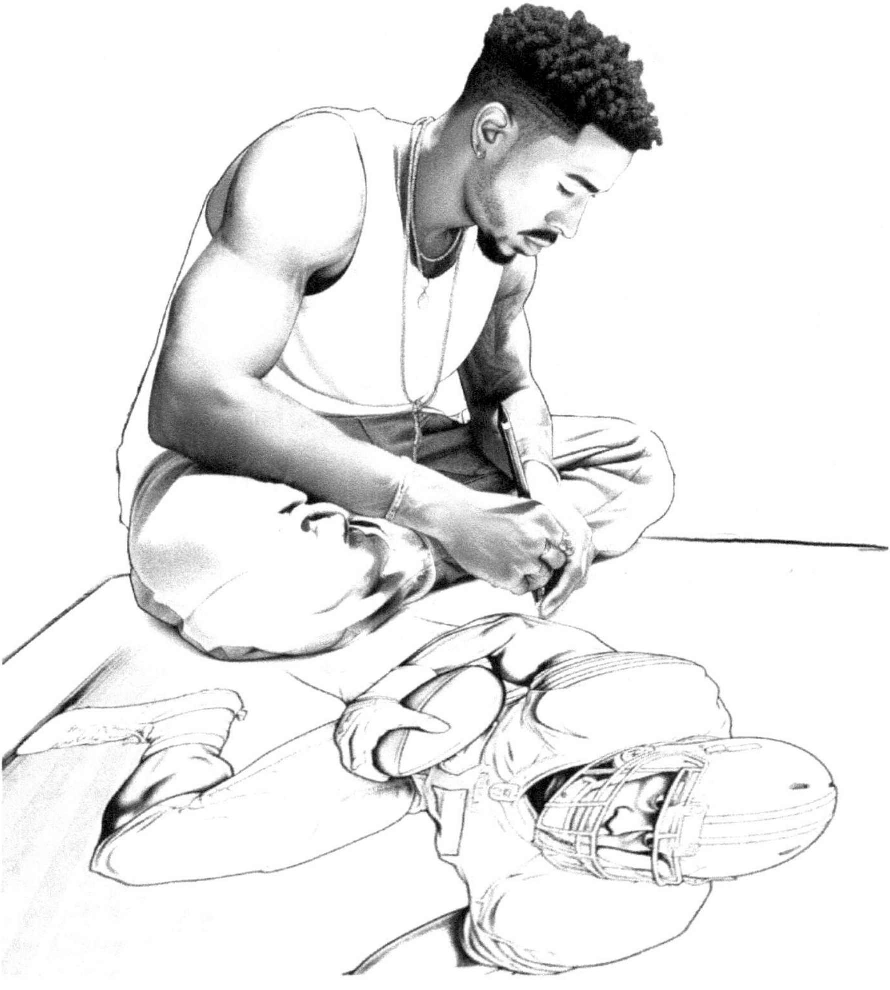

CHAPTER 15

MASTERS FOR HURTS

Success is usually graded by going viral and making lots of money. It's easy to forget that success can also be measured by another value—morals and giving back. It should be a way to remind yourself that being genuine and kind is a simple way to brighten someone else's day and create important memories. Also, it is a beautiful way to build character and to leave a positive impact on others. How great would it be if your peers knew you as a kind, generous and positive person? Maybe some people have doubts about you, or perhaps you've let your need to fit in and be popular (or hidden) prevent you from achieving your destiny or making connections with other classmates.

Why do coincidences happen? What is it about certain moments coming together at the right moment that makes one believe? Fate is a magical thing. Take the story of two young brothers from Louisiana who have admired Jalen Hurts, Philadelphia Eagles quarterback, from a distance (on television and via social media.). Before the school year started, one brother had a special request, a Jalen Hurts backpack, because he was motivated by how hard Jalen played the game and how brave he was even though he was traded to another team. In that young boy's mind, that attitude makes a champion. Unfortunately, no matter how hard the young man's mother looked, she couldn't find the right backpack anywhere, so she made a backpack she was sure her son would love, and he did. Jalen found out about it and wrote a tweet. Would you believe Jalen was inspired to thank the young man by creating a backpack to honor the kid's faith in him? In this moment, Hurts made a kid's dream come true and remained a beacon of positivity and kindness.

Jalen Hurts has said that he constantly pushes for intriguing and new ways to prove doubters wrong. He uses doubt to motivate him to set harder, more complex goals and then achieve them. Since being drafted in 2020, he has already collected a ton of honors, like playing in the championship game and being the youngest ever quarterback in history to accomplish this with the Philadelphia Eagles. Even though his team didn't win, he had an epic championship performance with over 300 passing yards and a touchdown—that's something to celebrate. Also, he has tried his hand at a bit of acting, received his master's degree in Human Relations from the University of Oklahoma, and is leading the way by being one of the few elite superstars to have all-female management—inspired by his mom who pursued higher education while juggling her career and raising Jalen and his siblings.

The Philadelphia Eagles' young quarterback isn't satisfied after having an impressive breakout year and a $255 million contract extension. He is committed to constantly improving himself and is focused on being the best he can be, concentrating on what he can control rather than external factors. Hurts' commitment and focus on his craft impresses his coaches and they are confident that his work ethic and grit will help him continue to smash record after record. In his second season as a starter, Hurts threw for 3,701 yards, had 22 passing touchdowns, rushed for 760 yards with 13 rushing scores, and he was nominated for a Most Valuable Player (MVP) and an Offensive Player of the Year award.

So, just circling back to the moral of Hurts' story. When you push yourself, who knows what you can achieve? Will you be the next Jalen Hurts and use the doubts of others to motivate you to be the best you can be?

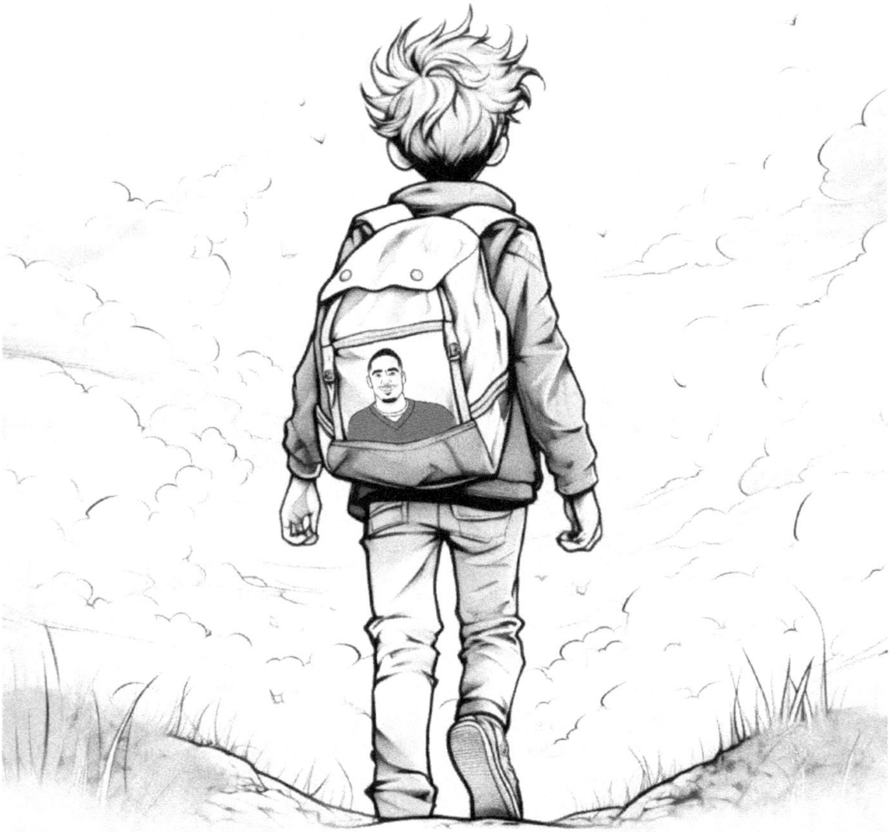

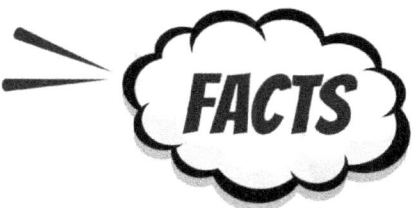

1. The only NFL team without last names on their jerseys is the Chicago Bears.

2. The 1966 Washington Redskins-New York Giants game was the NFL's highest-scoring game without overtime.

3. The Buffalo Bills are the first club to reach the Super Bowl four times (1990–1993) without winning.

4. In 2000, Tom Brady was picked in the sixth round (199th overall), one of the biggest draft bargains ever.

5. The first Super Bowl overtime was Super Bowl LI in 2017 between the Patriots and Falcons.

CHAPTER 16

A PERFECT MIRACLE IN MIAMI

Before their rise to fame, the Miami Dolphins struggled to succeed—would you believe it? From 1966 to 1969, they recorded four consecutive devastating losing seasons in their early years. However, in 1970, a significant change occurred when the Dolphins transitioned to the NFL, and they made a bold move in an attempt to better their team. They hired the legendary Don Shula as their head coach, luring him away from the Baltimore Colts.

The Dolphins' defense, famously known as the "No-Name Defense," played a pivotal role in the perfect season. The Dolphins earned their unique nickname because they lacked any big-name famous stars. Yet, at the same time, they consistently outperformed opponents. The journey to perfection was undoubtedly a bumpy road for the 1972 Dolphins, who faced many challenges in close games, unpredictable twists, and tests of their determination. Several games pushed this team to the limit, including matchups against the Minnesota Vikings, the Buffalo Bills, the playoff showdown with the Cleveland Browns, and the Divisional Championship Game against the Pittsburgh Steelers. Despite the better regular-season record, the Dolphins had to travel to Pittsburgh because of the playoff format at the time (in modern times, Pittsburgh would've traveled to Miami), forcing the Dolphins to feel like the underdogs in this situation. The game even started with the Steelers taking an early lead but as the game wound down, in a moment of inspiration, the punter executed a fake punt run, gaining almost 40 yards on the opponents, then a touchdown pass tied the game. Then coach Don Shula made a surprising halftime decision, switching quarterbacks, and paving the way for the Dolphins to take an unexpected yet brilliant win.

The grand finale was Super Bowl VII, in 1973, where the Dolphins faced off against the Washington Football Team (formerly known as the Redskins.) Just like the divisional game, the Dolphins were once again considered the underdogs, pushing the players to focus and be determined. They had to prove themselves despite the odds. While the Dolphins pulled off a victory to cap off the perfect season, it was marred by a play called "Garo's Gaffe." Dolphins kicker

Garo Yepremian's missed field goal attempt resulted in a touchdown for the Redskins. Why bring it up? Well, the impulsiveness of "Garo's Gaffe" could've cost the Dolphins the championship and put an end to the perfect season. Once I tell you a bit more about it, you'll understand why it's a top Championship Fail Play.

So, let's recap: Washington's defensive tackle blocked the field goal attempt; as the ball started bouncing away, Garo saw his chance, grabbed it, and took off running. It may have been better if he just fell and stopped the clock, but Garo was determined to try. Anyway, things kept going downhill, and Garo became more desperate with every minute, it looked like the kicker was going to dropkick his way through the opposition when Garo threw the ball. What could go wrong? The throw. Garo, realizing his mistake, started panicking and tried to bat the ball into the sidelines, and guess what? That didn't work either. The ball landed in the hands of a Washington cornerback, who ran it in for the touchdown. Luckily, it all ended well; Garo's (and the Dolphins) prayers were answered, and they won the game.

It has been over 50 years since the 1973 Super Bowl, where the NFL champion team for the 1972 season would be decided—and the Miami Dolphins came out on top. The team enjoyed their perfect season, and while many teams have tried, none have been able to achieve this kind of incredible accomplishment. So, what lessons can we learn from this? Firstly, it is a testament to what can be achieved with a little excellence, consistency, and sheer determination. Here, excellence for the 1972 Dolphins was more about being their best. Each player embraced a tireless commitment to being the best they could be, and winning came along for the ride. Let this motivate and inspire you to be open to solutions and have the courage to be resilient and try new things to achieve your goals.

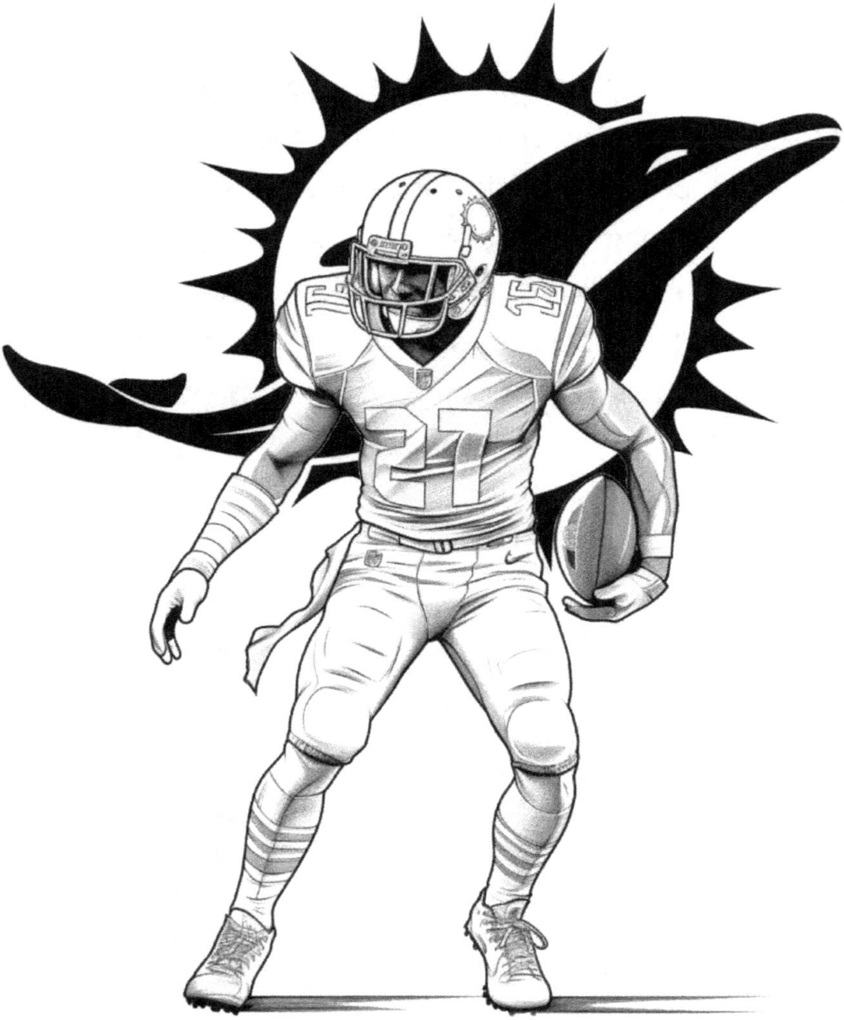

CHAPTER 17

FOR #3, WITH LOVE

In January 2023, Damar Hamlin suffered an injury on the field while playing for the Buffalo Bills. The game, which was against the Cincinnati Bengals, was soon called off following his injury. Damar Hamlin's scary experience on the football field that day reminds us all that inner strength is not about avoiding challenges but facing them head on. One key lesson from Hamlin's journey is the strength that comes from having a good support system around you. The outpouring of love, prayers, and encouragement from the community in Buffalo (and throughout the football community) during his recovery shows how important it is to have the support of people who care for us. Everyone was rallying behind Hamlin and hoping for a speedy recovery. It is nice to know that when challenges seem impossible, or we have doubts, we can turn to our friends, family, and even strangers to guide us through the rough times.

Hamlin's admirable ability to maintain a positive outlook despite misfortune teaches us a valuable lesson: A positive attitude can drive us forward in life and that digging deep and focusing on being strong is not just a comeback but an intentional reaction to overcome challenging times. We can be positive and focus on using difficult times as opportunities for growth, and we learn to practice gratitude and focus on being hopeful.

Months later, in a heartfelt letter, Damar Hamlin expressed his deep gratitude and admiration for the Buffalo community and the overwhelming amount of support he received. In his letter, Hamlin described how much he admires the community who united in harmony to wish him a quick and healthy recovery. Also, the letter shares how special Damar felt and how much it meant to him and his family that the people of Buffalo took the time to show their love and support of the city that touched them. What he appreciated the most was reading the cards, letters, admiring the artwork from school-aged kids, hearing about how others prayed for him, and seeing people wearing his jersey number. It truly shows how dedicated their fans, and the whole community, are to this team. All of this motivated Hamlin to get better and reminded him how blessed he was to have the chance to continue giving back to the community that showed up for him during a dark time. The letter thanked Buffalo for its ongoing love and support, which he felt played a significant role in his healing process.

Damar Hamlin's journey is one of extraordinary strength and positivity. In the locker room, Hamlin is famous for his positivity and for bringing an endearing, joyful spirit that motivates anyone around him. It's incredible and admirable how this same energy was returned to him when he was the one needing positivity. Hamlin is grateful that the people of Buffalo have welcomed him, and he is thankful to the city that inspires him to keep praying, loving, and aspiring for greatness. His resilience in the face of adversity is striking; he never let personal challenges affect his demeanor or commitment to the team.

Bills' quarterback, Josh Allen, told a story about a visit to see Hamlin after the severe injury Hamlin suffered. He recalled that Hamlin's first concern was not about himself but more about who won the game—a tiny example of Hamlin's team spirit and selflessness.

While the football community hoped and prayed for Damar, people began donating to the foundation Damar created, The Chasing M's foundation, and through online campaigns, raised over 8 million dollars. The foundation supports community-based goals via toy drives, back-to-school initiatives, and kids' camps.

Damar Hamlin's journey shows that when you care about your community, your community can and often rallies around you when you least expect it. Isn't that inspiring? No matter who we are, if we care, we can make a difference, whether for ourselves or those close to us, or it can inspire many lives. Think about how you could make a difference in your community. For his community efforts, Hamlin received an important award, called NFLPA Alan Page Community Award—an award given to players who improve their communities locally and worldwide.

Bouncing back from hard times is an important skill—it helps to give us drive, focus, and determination to overcome obstacles, no matter how difficult or impossible they seem. Hamlin's story is a reminder that it's normal to suffer through hard times, but as long as you bounce back, you're not letting the hardship win.

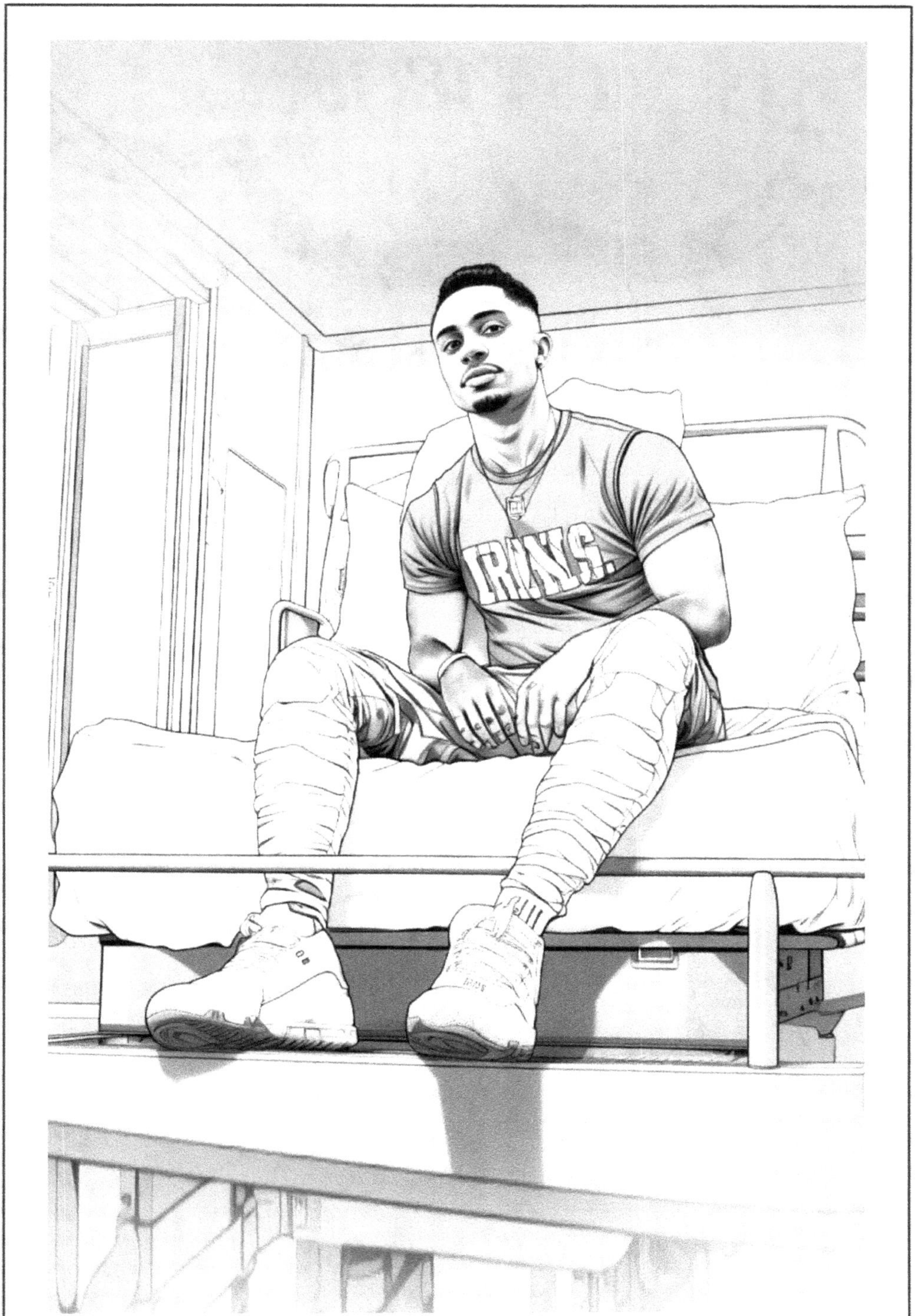

CHAPTER 18

THE ICY (ICE) BOWL

You'll notice plenty of closed (and covered) stadiums in today's game, so you'd think it'd be easier to avoid those bone-chilling game days. But nope, they're still very much a thing of the present. One January day in 1994, the Bills faced the LA (Los Angeles) Raiders; the day started at a 'warm' 0 °F degrees before the chill quickly set in, and temperatures fell to -32 °F—that's a drastic difference. The Minnesota Vikings faced a similar fate in 2016 against the Seattle Seahawks, -6 °F and a wind chill of -25 °F; the poor Vikings didn't stand a chance in these weather conditions. Their kicker missed a 27-yard field goal and only managed 183 yards of offense during the game. Over 40 years ago, in 1982, the San Diego Chargers played the Cincinnati Bengals and soldiered through four quarters against a wind chill of a whopping -59 °F.

As cold as these games were, they were still mid and couldn't even begin to compare to The Icy Bowl of 1967—a divisional championship match starring the Dallas Cowboys and the Green Bay Packers. The day before the big game, everyone enjoyed the relatively mild 20 °F or so weather; the weather soon did a 180 and took a sharp turn, plunging the over the 50,000-plus fans, coaching staff, and players into frigid -13 °F of relentless cold with a wind chill that was as low as -48 °F. Each team played their best to find a victory on Lambeau Field's icy, frozen surface—call it ice hockey at this point, am I right? Each team worked together to stay sharp, focused, and warm, but the Packers ended up emerging victorious on this icy day.

Going through extreme situations may not be something you can prepare for, but that doesn't mean you shouldn't try to push yourself—you never know what you can accomplish. Why is pushing yourself to your limits an important and valuable experience? Battling through hard times and overcoming challenges can inspire you and move you toward being adaptable and create moments that allow you to be free to leave your stamp on the world. Facing your fears and weaknesses and overcoming challenging moments tests you in various ways, hopefully letting you realize that you have the power to be stronger than you thought was possible.

Who knows, maybe sharing how you pushed through a tough situation that you didn't think you could manage may give you a well-needed confidence boost, or perhaps it can inspire someone else to try their best. No matter what, use the new knowledge you've gained by embracing these challenging moments and pushing yourself toward a journey of growth and change. Just remember that difficult situations can force you to think outside of the box and be able to recognize and attempt to discover creative ways to solve complex problems. Remember this, adapting to change can be a good thing so take it in your stride.

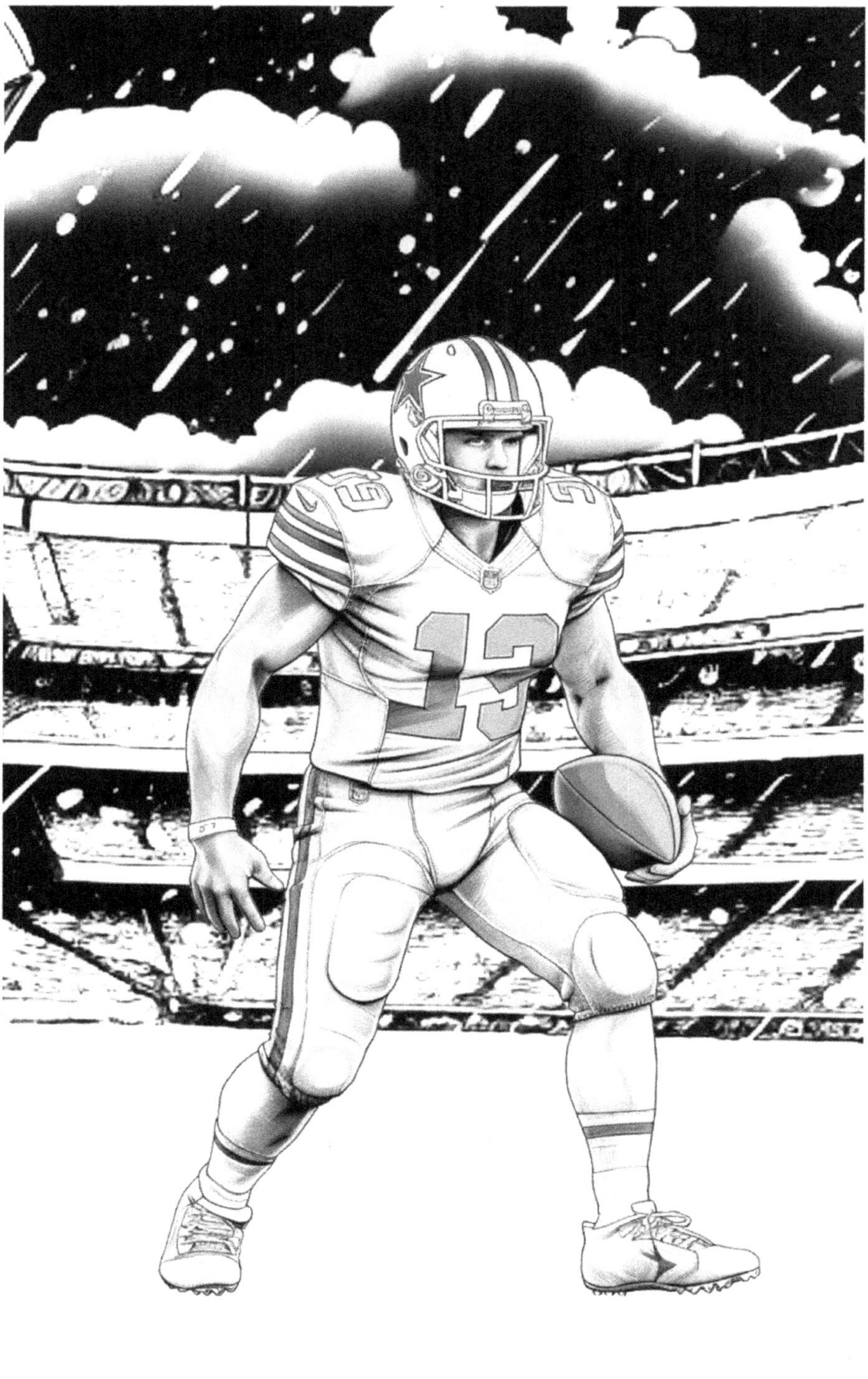

CHAPTER 19

JUMPIN' LAMBEAU, LAMBEAU LEAP

Yes, we're back again at Lambeau Field for this inspirational tale, the home of a celebration you should know about—call it a leap of faith, I suppose. Maybe returning to this place is just another way to bring up the icy conditions and how coincidental it is that the players have time to come up with unique ways to celebrate with their fans. Maybe the cold inspires creativity; who knows?

Let's introduce you to LeRoy Butler and see how a spur-of-the-moment idea became an honored tradition that is well-loved by the Green Bay Packers and their dedicated fans to this day. During a touchdown play, Butler was sprinting along the sidelines to the end zone when a fun idea hit him. As he crossed the line and scored the touchdown, the ball fell out of his hands; Butler pointed to the crowd and asked them to catch him and just like that, Butler goes up a few feet and is caught by a few of the fans in the crowd who quickly shouted words of encouragement and were delighted to have such a close-up interaction with an NFL star. Within seconds, the moment is over, and the game continues. Just like that, a treasured moment is over and lost in time.

Butler's spontaneous leap of faith didn't go viral, as things couldn't back then, with no highlight reels to capture this incredible moment, but it planted a seed, a leap of faith that came to be called the Lambeau Leap. Let's dive into the origin story. Butler created the Leap, but as the story goes, another player took the idea, made it popular, and ran with it. His name was Robert Brooks.

Brooks played for the Packers from 1992 to 1998; he was a favorite target of QB Brett Favre and scored over 30 TDs during his time with the team. After crossing into the end zone, Brooks often leaped into the stands, popularizing the Lambeau Leap; he may have written a song about his celebration (but that's a story for another day).

Besides Butler and Brooks, other players have taken the famous Leap, too! Some popular ones are back in 2006 when Favre scored a rushing TD that gave the Packers a 21-point lead and leaped into the crowd after celebrating with his teammates. Legendary QB Aaron Rodgers has several Lambeau Leaps under his belt. In 2016, during a stellar game where he threw for over 340 yards with five TDs, he leaped after a 6-yard TD play in the second quarter of that game. (An honorable mention for a hilarious failed attempt goes to John Kuhn; back in 2014, he couldn't get any air to scale the wall; instead, he "celebrated" by landing next to the wall—each to their own, I suppose).

Acting out (or following through on) spontaneous ideas takes a lot of courage—it's easy to keep your head down and follow the same old rules and concepts. We all feel like that sometimes. But why is that? Sometimes, we can let our fears force us to be complacent and unwilling to try out new ideas. Don't be shy, and it's crucial to express and share your thoughts and ideas with others—it's incredible to watch what happens when it's a collaborative effort. When people work together, different perspectives start developing and leave lasting impressions, especially when it comes to sharing and expanding upon traditions. You can build on the sense of community, provide opportunities to share their experiences and build stronger bonds with those around you. And who knows what you can become when you're brave enough to take a leap of faith? Maybe you'll create an iconic Lambeau Leap-like tradition of your own.

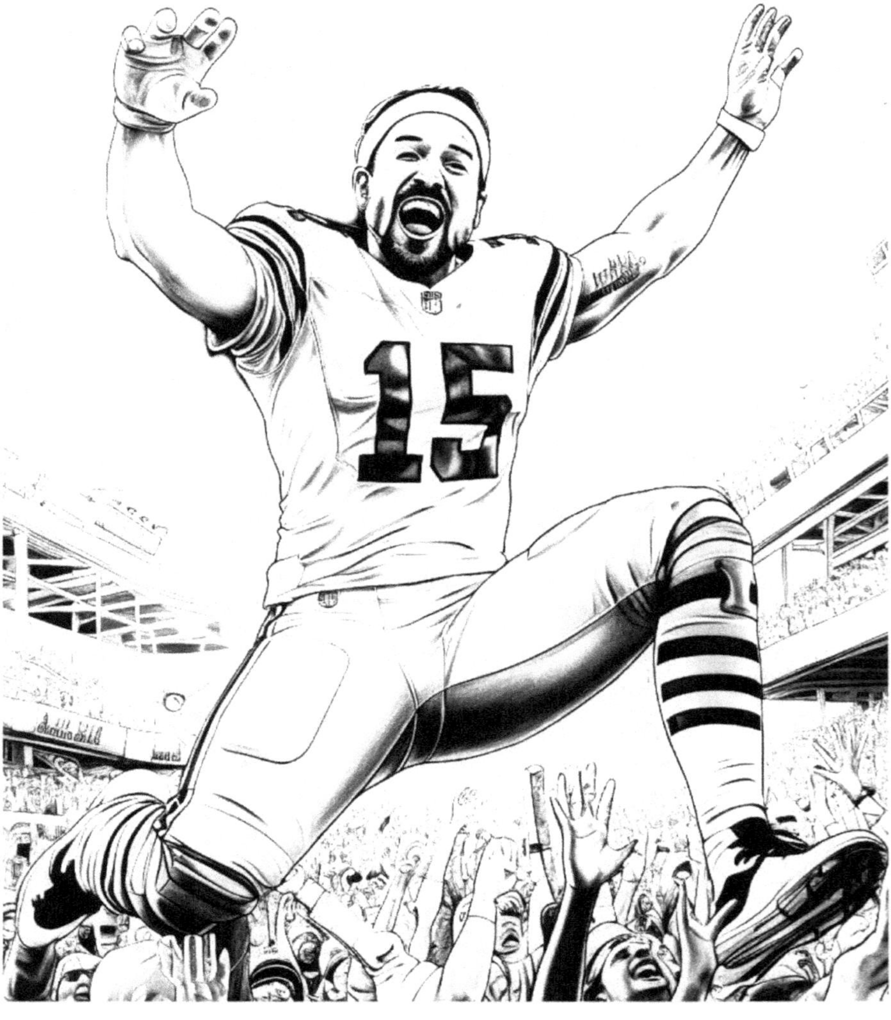

CHAPTER 20

A FAIL MARY—WHICH CALL SHOULD'VE STOOD?

Our last story hails from a suspenseful Monday night in 2012. Two refs, two different calls. Who will get the final say?

Referee number one said interception. Referee number two raised his arms in the air—a touchdown! How is it that they both saw different things? We may never know.

Anyway, the ruling on the field stood. Two rulings were called, and only one can stand. Why did this Hail Mary Play spark a controversy? And a new hilarious nickname, Fail Mary.

The Seattle Seahawks were just seconds away from losing a game to the Green Bay Packers, down by three points. Seahawks fans were preparing for disappointment, and Packers fans were anticipating a night of celebrations ahead. Seahawks quarterback Russell Wilson desperately launched the football in hopes someone could get it into the end zone for the win—it's always worth a shot, right? A Seahawks wide receiver may have been a little rough during a shoving match with a Packers cornerback; the play should've drawn a penalty or at least a review. It didn't. As the scrambling on the field continues, Golden Tate (Seahawks) and M. D. Jennings (Packers) are in the corner of the end zone; both hit the ground and have possession of the ball.

Now that you're all caught up with the last vital moments of the game, this whirlwind of confusion left the referees stumped. Which call stands? This decision was fueled by pressure; the stats of each team lay in the referees' hands. After further review, the call that stood was in favor of the Seahawks. The next day, the League reviewed the game and admitted mistakes. Tate's shove should have been called offensive pass interference in an earlier play. If it had, the following play between the players wouldn't have happened, so the debate about whether Tate or Jennings caught the ball also wouldn't have happened, and the Packers would have won the game! How did the referees get so mixed up on the rules? As it turns out, the referees were on loan from local high school and college leagues.

Surely you've heard the saying rules are meant to be broken, right? We talked about how great it can be to follow your dreams or share an idea everyone likes. Why bother with rules? Especially when things are going your way—you may think it seems pointless. Maybe you're scared about the consequences or don't see the effects because you want to fit in. It's hard to ignore the urge to bend the rules a bit and deal with the consequences later or never. Remember, being respectful and a good listener can go a long way to helping you understand the "why" behind the rules. Every rule has its reason, whether it's to keep you safe or make sure everyone is treated fairly.

Haven't you noticed before that when rules are unclear and inconsistently actioned, you're more uneasy dealing with feelings or a sense of unfairness (bias) and easily frustrated? Maybe the instructions for your math test were unclear, or perhaps you tried getting away with not doing chores properly? Things usually backfire—that's why rules and clear instructions are always laid out. Respecting boundaries, being accountable, and following rules can help maintain trust and encourage competitiveness.

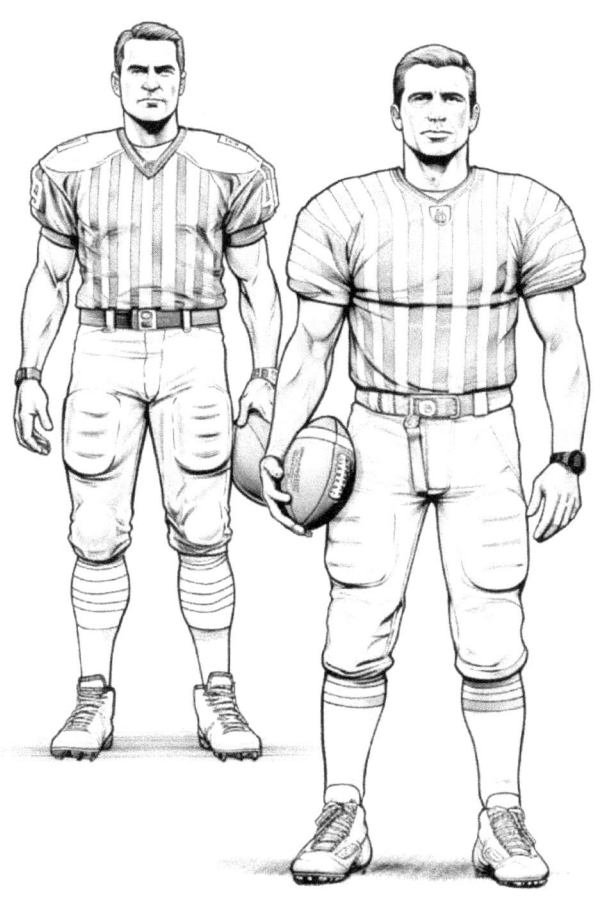

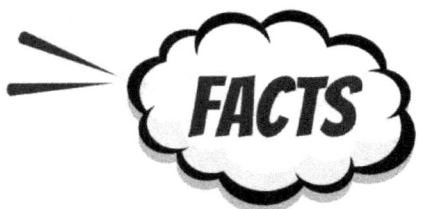

FACTS

1. Jerry Rice, a legendary wide receiver, trained by catching bricks to strengthen his hands.

2. Marshawn Lynch loves Skittles, so supporters would toss them on the field to celebrate his touchdowns.

3. The typical NFL game lasts 3 hours and 12 minutes, but the ball is only in play for 11 minutes.

4. The NFL's first costumed mascot was Billy Buffalo of the Buffalo Bills.

5. With 14 jersey numbers retired, the Chicago Bears have the most in NFL history.

CONCLUSION

So, after all these American football tales you've read in detail, what have we learned from these short stories of triumphant success, funny mishaps, and epic comebacks? The answer is... we've learned quite a lot! Let's have a recap;

Thanks to Bernie Kosar's incredible twist of fate, we've unraveled that there's no need to be so hard on yourself when things go wrong. Making mistakes is perfectly normal, but what's most important is that we get back up and learn from them. A little mistake isn't the end of the world, but just an opportunity to learn something new about yourself. The Pittsburgh Steelers taught us that, as cliche as it may sound, practice really does make perfect. Have faith in your abilities and continue to work hard to get what you deserve—your commitment to bettering yourself will always pay off.

Jon Dorenbos' iconically magic America's Got Talent expedition showed us that multiple talents we possess can come together to provide a beautiful blend of fun and creativity with strength and passion. Other life lessons have reinforced the value of listening carefully to instructions and the reason why rules are in place or that a little bit of creativity and imagination can provide remarkable results

Oh, and how could we forget, Mac Jones' delightful fascination with freezing temperatures, the cold air, and his own breath trails.

Whatever you take from these stories, I'm sure you've learned some valuable lessons and, hopefully, got a good laugh out of some of these tales. And, for one last laugh, may I share a pun? It's truly been a touchdown of wisdom and life lessons.

Football Short Stories for Kids Touchdown Tales: Funny Mishaps and Inspirational Moments from the World of American Football has provided you with some incredible recollections of American football history with valuable lessons for kids.

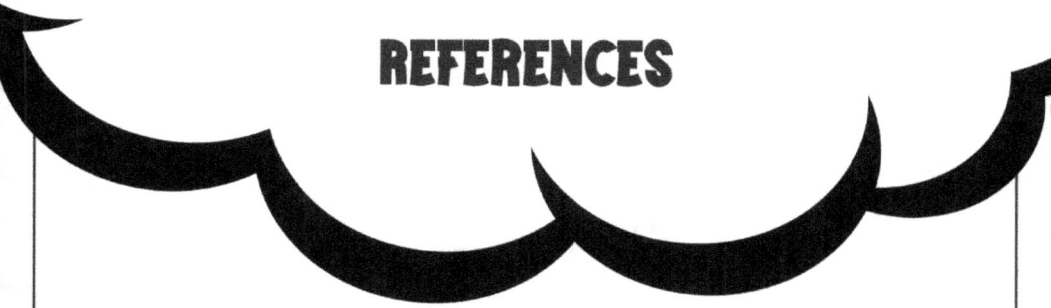

REFERENCES

Albert , D. (2022, January 16). Mac Jones goes viral for funny moment with Josh McDaniels on sideline. Yardbarker. https://www.yardbarker.com/nfl/articles/mac_jones_goes_viral_for_funny_moment_with_josh_mcdaniels_on_sideline/s1_127_36998153

Baker, G. (2013, November 27). Coolest things NFL players have done for fans. Bleacher Report. https://bleacherreport.com/articles/1855772-coolest-things-nfl-players-have-done-for-fans

Branch, J. (2010, January 8). Chad Ochocinco, the N.F.L. leader in attention (Published 2010). *The New York Times.* https://www.nytimes.com/2010/01/09/sports/football/09ochocinco.html

Burke, C. (2021, August 4). Megatron memories: Calvin Johnson rewatches the greatest moments from a Hall of Fame career. The Athletic. https://theathletic.com/2731041/2021/08/04/megatron-memories-calvin-johnson-rewatches-the-greatest-moments-from-a-hall-of-fame-career/

Callahan, R. (2008, December 6). Top 10 NFL touchdown celebrations of all time. Bleacher Report. https://bleacherreport.com/articles/89902-top-10-nfl-touchdown-celebrations-of-all-time

Camenker, J. (2022, September 15). "Lambeau Leap" origin, explained: How LeRoy Butler started Packers' long-standing tradition and celebration. Www.sportingnews.com. https://www.sportingnews.com/ca/nfl/news/lambeau-leap-packers-origin-leroy-butler/objj7fup6xljtvyq4tazpjrh

CBC Kids News. (2023, January 6). NFL player Damar Hamlin speaking again after cardiac arrest during game. CBC Kids News. https://www.cbc.ca/kidsnews/post/nfl-player-damar-hamlin-recovering-after-cardiac-arrest

A complete overview of Tom Brady's New England Patriots Career. (2023). Www.sportskeeda.com. https://www.sportskeeda.com/nfl/tom-bradys-new-england-patriots-career

Crawford, R. (2023). The Most Surprising Super Bowl Wins of the 21st Century — The Sporting Blog. Thesporting.blog. https://thesporting.blog/blog/most-surprising-super-bowl-wins-of-the-21st-century-nfl

Cudahy, M. (2023, September 7). NFL returns: Watch these heartwarming videos from this past offseason. WESH. https://www.wesh.com/article/human-interest-stories-from-nfl-offseason/45038649

D'Abate, M. (2023, February 5). Patriots, Tom Brady 28-3 Super Bowl LI Comeback: Still Legendary. Sports Illustrated New England Patriots News, Analysis and More. https://www.si.com/nfl/patriots/news/new-england-patriots-super-bowl-li-comeback-tom-brady-james-white-julian-edelman-movie

D'Amato, G. (2017, December 28). The Ice Bowl, 50 years later: An oral history of the Packers-Cowboys 1967 NFL Championship Game. Milwaukee Journal Sentinel; Milwaukee. https://www.jsonline.com/story/sports/nfl/packers/2017/12/28/ice-bowl-50-years-later-oral-history-packers-cowboys-1967-nfl-championship-game/962212001/

Daniels, M. (2022, January 3). Mark Daniels: Patriots' Mac Jones is one of the best rookie quarterbacks of all-time. The Providence Journal. https://www.providencejournal.com/story/sports/nfl/patriots/2022/01/03/new-england-patriots-mac-jones-one-of-the-best-rookie-quarterbacks-in-nfl-history/9074297002/

DaSilva, C. (2016, March 8). The 10 craziest stats from Calvin Johnson's illustrious career. FOX Sports. https://www.foxsports.com/stories/nfl/the-10-craziest-stats-from-calvin-johnsons-illustrious-career

DeArdo, B. (2023, May 19). Jim Brown dies at 87: Ranking the greatest rookie seasons in NFL history; where the Cleveland great fits. CBSSports.com. https://www.cbssports.com/nfl/news/jim-brown-dies-at-87-ranking-the-greatest-rookie-seasons-in-nfl-history-where-the-cleveland-great-fits/#:~:text=Sayers

Diaz, G. (2018, September 19). The day Golden Tate "caught" Russell Wilson's last-second Hail Mary. Andscape. https://andscape.com/features/the-day-golden-tate-caught-russell-wilsons-last-second-hail-mary/

Didinger, R. (2019, September 21). Didinger: Philly Special symbolic of Eagles' drive to Super Bowl Championship. Www.philadelphiaeagles.com. https://www.philadelphiaeagles.com/news/didinger-philly-special-symbolic-of-eagles-drive-to-super-bowl-championship

Dozier, A. (2023, February 27). How the Record Sale of "The Sugar Shack" Made Ernie Barnes the Comeback Kid. Artsy. https://www.artsy.net/article/artsy-editorial-record-sale-the-sugar-shack-made-ernie-barnes-comeback-kid

Dye, N. (2023, February 13). Jason Kelce Says He and Brother Travis "Talked More This Year Than" They Have "Since College." Peoplemag. https://people.com/sports/super-bowl-2023-jason-kelce-brother-travis-talked-more-this-year-than-since-college/

Eagles QB Jalen Hurts says, "There's a thrill in not being satisfied" - CBS Philadelphia. (2023, July 6). Www.cbsnews.com. https://www.cbsnews.com/philadelphia/news/eagles-qb-jalen-hurts-says-theres-a-thrill-in-not-being-satisfied-2/

Eidell, L. (2023, April 19). Travis Kelce and Jason Kelce: Everything to Know About the NFL Brothers. Peoplemag. https://people.com/sports/all-about-brothers-travis-kelce-jason-kelce/

ESPN.com. (2023). Mac Jones Stats, News, Bio. ESPN. https://www.espn.com/nfl/player/_/id/4241464/mac-jones

Ferguson, A. (2010, October 13). You Can Dance If You Wanna; The Most Memorable TD Celebrations in NFL History. Bleacher Report. https://bleacherreport.com/

articles/490071-you-can-dance-if-you-wanna-the-most-memorable-td-celebrations-in-nfl-history

50 Years Ago: The "Ice Bowl." (2017). Nflcommunications.com. https://nflcommunications.com/Pages/50-Years-Ago--The-Ice-Bowl.aspx

Gandhi, S. (2021, November 16). Where did these NFL nicknames come from? *SI Kids: Sports News for Kids, Kids Games and More.* https://www.sikids.com/nfl/nfl-nicknames#:~:text=While%20the%20origin%20is%20a

Getzenberg, A. (2021, October 18). How the Buffalo Bills pulled off the greatest comeback in NFL history. ESPN.com. https://www.espn.com/nfl/story/_/id/32405466/how-buffalo-bills-pulled-greatest-comeback-nfl-history

Greatest Comebacks in NFL History | Pro Football Hall of Fame. (2021). Pfhof. https://www.profootballhof.com/football-history/greatest-comebacks-in-nfl-history/

Gregory , S. (2023, September 13). Jalen Hurts is fueled by the doubters. Time. https://time.com/6312770/jalen-hurts-interview-time-100-next/

Hamlin, D. (2023, September 19). Damar Hamlin: Thank you, Buffalo. Reader's Digest. https://www.rd.com/article/damar-hamlin-thank-you-buffalo/

Heidinger, G. (2023, January 7). "Far more than just a football player" | How Damar Hamlin's warrior spirit and giving nature is an inspiration to many. Www.buffalobills.com. https://www.buffalobills.com/news/far-more-than-just-a-football-player-how-damar-hamlin-s-warrior-spirit-and-givin

Heifetz, D. (2021, August 30). *What's More Important in NFL Quarterback Development: Nature or Nurture?* The Ringer. https://www.theringer.com/nfl/2021/8/30/22647741/nfl-quarterbacks-nature-nurture-trevor-lawrence-zach-wilson-trey-lance-justin-fields

Hightower, K. (2023, August 3). Trash talking and playful, Mac Jones makes having fun a priority this season. USA TODAY. https://www.usatoday.com/story/sports/nfl/2023/08/03/trash-talking-and-playful-mac-jones-makes-having-fun-a-priority-this-season/70522560007/

Horton, C. (2012, January 30). The most surprising Super Bowl winners ever. Bleacher Report. https://bleacherreport.com/articles/1046203-the-most-surprising-super-bowl-winners-ever

Hunt, D. J. (2023, August 3). Tom Brady: Career retrospective. Yardbarker. https://www.yardbarker.com/nfl/articles/tom_brady_career_retrospective/s1__37630494#slide_2

Iyer, V. (2022, December 15). Who caught the Immaculate Reception? Explaining the legendary 1972 Steelers vs. Raiders play and controversy. Www.sportingnews.com. https://www.sportingnews.com/ca/nfl/news/immaculate-reception-steelers-play-nfl-history/nyvilvqarxxfk28eexy1dnlo

Jeremiah, D. (2022, January 14). NFL rookie rankings: Ja'Marr Chase, Micah Parsons headline top 25 after transcendent regular season. NFL.com. https://www.nfl.com/news/nfl-rookie-rankings-ja-marr-chase-micah-parsons-headline-top-25-after-transcende

Jones, L. H. (2015, February 5). Nick Foles' trick-play TD catch in Super Bowl was true "Philly Special." USA TODAY. https://www.usatoday.com/story/sports/nfl/eagles/2018/02/05/nick-foles-trick-play-td-catch-super-bowl-philadelphia-eagles/306204002/

Jr, M. F. (2018, February 15). Philadelphia Eagles Super Bowl win fast tracks movie on Long Snapper/Magician Jon Dorenbos. Deadline. https://deadline.com/2018/02/jon-dorenbos-philadelphia-eagles-super-bowl-movie-mike-tollin-americas-got-talent-1202288378/

Kasabian, P. (2023, September 18). Damar Hamlin, Lids HD launch "Bills Mafia" collection; money to be donated to charity. Bleacher Report. https://bleacherreport.com/articles/10089905-damar-hamlin-lids-hd-launch-bills-mafia-collection-money-to-be-donated-to-charity

Kessler, M. (2019, December 13). Magic, football And tragedy: The story of Jon Dorenbos. Www.wbur.org. https://www.wbur.org/onlyagame/2019/12/13/jon-dorenbos-magician-eagles-nfl-book

Koons, Z. (2023, February 12). Look: Donna Kelce shares amazing Super Bowl gameday outfit. Sports Illustrated. https://www.si.com/extra-mustard/2023/02/12/donna-kelce-shares-amazing-super-bowl-gameday-outfit#:~:text=Her%20multicolored%20jacket%20was%20split

Kostos, N. (2013, January 25). The top 10 Super Bowls in NFL history. Bleacher Report. https://bleacherreport.com/articles/1500765-the-top-10-super-bowls-of-all-time

Lazar, E. (2023, January 11). Season review: Evaluating Mac Jones's second season and how the Patriots move forward at quarterback. Www.patriots.com. https://www.patriots.com/news/season-review-evaluating-mac-jones-second-season-and-how-the-patriots-move-for

Lazarus Caplan, A. (2023, February 13). Travis Kelce gets emotional after beating big brother Jason in Super Bowl: "It's a weird feeling." Peoplemag. https://people.com/sports/super-bowl-2023-travis-kelce-emotional-after-beating-big-brother-jason/

Marlow, D. (2023, January 30). The 10 best NFL siblings of all time took brotherly love to the gridiron. FanBuzz. https://fanbuzz.com/nfl/best-nfl-siblings/

Marvi, R. (2022, February 3). The life and career of Andre Johnson (complete story). Pro Football History. https://www.profootballhistory.com/andre-johnson/

McDermott, M. (2019, February 4). Play of the Super Bowl: Jason McCourty's end zone pass break up. Pats Pulpit. https://www.patspulpit.com/2019/2/4/18210180/2019-super-bowl-play-of-the-game-new-england-patriots-los-angeles-rams-jason-mccourty-brandin-cooks

McPherson, C. (2020, August 19). The story of Jalen Hurts, a young fan, and an unbelievable coincidence. Www.philadelphiaeagles.com. https://www.philadelphiaeagles.com/news/the-story-of-jalen-hurts-a-young-fan-and-an-unbelievable-coincidence

McVey, R. (2023, February 1). 25 greatest quarterbacks in NFL History. AthlonSports.com. https://athlonsports.com/nfl/25-greatest-quarterbacks-nfl-history-2016

Neumann, S. (2023, May 15). Eagles QB Jalen Hurts continues to "be the best version of myself" as he earns master's degree. Peoplemag. https://people.com/sports/jalen-hurts-eagles-qb-earns-masters-degree/#:~:text=%22I%20Know%20Momma%20Proud%20Of

NFL.com. (2023a). Brothers in the NFL. NFL.com. https://www.nfl.com/photos/brothers-in-the-nfl-0ap3000000925746

NFL.com. (2023b). Greatest comebacks in NFL history. NFL.com. https://www.nfl.com/photos/greatest-comebacks-in-nfl-history-0ap3000000646081

Oguntola, B. (2022, October 21). 1972 Miami Dolphins – the perfect season 50th anniversary. Www.miamidolphins.com. https://www.miamidolphins.com/news/1972-miami-dolphins-the-perfect-season-50th-anniversary

Olson, T. (2022, December 21). 5 coldest NFL games in league history. Pro Football Network. https://www.profootballnetwork.com/coldest-games-in-nfl-history/

Oz, Dr. M., & Michaels, B. (2019). NFL 100. NFL.com. https://www.nfl.com/100/originals/100-greatest/plays-1

Picaro, C. (2022, December 19). The Lambeau Leap: An NFL tradition started by an unlikely player. FanBuzz. https://fanbuzz.com/nfl/first-lambeau-leap/

Powell, W. (2011, August 30). Ochocinco's top ten touchdown celebrations. Cincinnati Magazine. https://www.cincinnatimagazine.com/bengals/ochocincos-top-ten-touchdown-celebrations1/

Reed, J. (2013, October 27). Calvin Johnson nearly breaks NFL receiving record in thrilling win vs. Cowboys. Bleacher Report. https://bleacherreport.com/articles/1826930-calvin-johnson-nearly-breaks-nfl-receiving-record-in-thrilling-win-vs-cowboys

Riddle, R. (2014, January 27). Marshawn Lynch: The man behind beast mode. Bleacher Report. https://bleacherreport.com/articles/1938021-marshawn-lynch-the-man-behind-beastmode

Robinson, S. (2021, August 23). The greatest siblings in NFL history. Yardbarker. https://www.yardbarker.com/nfl/articles/the_greatest_siblings_in_nfl_history/s1__30603515

Robinson, S. (2023, August 20). The most unlikely Super Bowl teams. Yardbarker. https://www.yardbarker.com/nfl/articles/the_most_unlikely_super_bowl_teams_081823/s1__37199948#slide_1

Ryan, C. (2023, May 9). Mac Jones' former teammate shares story about Patriots QB's work ethic. Www.boston.com. https://www.boston.com/sports/new-england-patriots/2023/05/08/mac-jones-former-alabama-teammate-shares-story-about-patriots-qbs-work-ethic-in-college/

Scataglia, L. (2023, July 16). Patriots' QB Mac Jones is under historic pressure in the 2023 season. Musket Fire. https://musketfire.com/posts/patriots-qb-mac-jones-is-under-historic-pressure-in-the-2023-season-01h5fjdh7w89

Schuller, R. (2023, February 8). The Philly Special: What is it? The story behind the incredible "Philly Philly" Super Bowl trick play | DAZN News US. DAZN. https://www.dazn.com/

en-US/news/football/the-philly-special-what-is-it-the-story-behind-the-incredible-philly-philly-super-bowl-trick-play/12o7hceprvh8h1bhp8hu96sqke

Sherman, R. (2022, September 23). Ten years later, the failed lessons from the fail Mary. The Ringer. https://www.theringer.com/nfl/2022/9/23/23366808/fail-mary-nfl-anniversary-green-bay-packers-seattle-seahawks

Spadaro, D. (2023, May 15). Jalen Hurts on earning master's degree: "Nobody can take this away from me." Www.philadelphiaeagles.com. https://www.philadelphiaeagles.com/news/jalen-hurts-on-earning-masters-degree-nobody-can-take-this-away-from-me

Sutelan, E. (2023, February 5). Kelce vs. Kelce Bowl: 4 fun facts to know about NFL's first Super Bowl between brothers on field. Www.sportingnews.com. https://www.sportingnews.com/ca/nfl/news/kelce-vs-kelce-super-bowl-brothers/pvjnd7i6unxghezrv4dfxk85

Tanier, M. (2016, October 5). Urban Legends of the NFL: Did frightened refs stage the Immaculate Reception? Bleacher Report. https://bleacherreport.com/articles/2662252-urban-legends-of-the-nfl-did-frightened-refs-stage-the-immaculate-reception#:~:text=Officials%20were%20not%20certain%20whether

Thompson, D. (2023, August 9). Could this season be a mirror image of Mac Jones' rookie year in 2021? Musket Fire. https://musketfire.com/posts/could-this-season-be-a-mirror-image-of-mac-jones-rookie-year-in-2021-01h7bea8kwdr

Weber, B. (2009, April 30). Ernie Barnes, artist and athlete, dies at 70. *The New York Times*. https://www.nytimes.com/2009/04/30/arts/30barnes.html

Wertheim, J. (2022, October 24). Life story of Garo Yepremian, kicker for undefeated '72 Dolphins - Sports Illustrated. *Sports Illustrated*. https://www.si.com/nfl/2022/10/24/garo-yepremian-incredible-journey-beyond-super-bowl-blooper-daily-cover#

Wolfe, C. (2022, August 25). 1972 Miami Dolphins: The inside story of the only perfect season in NFL history. NFL.com. https://www.nfl.com/news/sidelines/1972-miami-dolphins-the-inside-story-of-the-only-perfect-season-in-nfl-history

Yuscavage, C. (2014, December 11). Marshawn Lynch explains meaning of "Beast Mode" in Most Marshawn Lynch way possible. Complex. https://www.complex.com/sports/a/chris-yuscavage/marshawn-lynch-seahawks-rb-explains-meaning-beast-mode

Zaldivar, G. (2012, December 4). Andre Johnson shows true meaning of Christmas, *drops $19 k on CPS gifts*. Bleacher Report. https://bleacherreport.com/articles/1433075-andre-johnson-shows-true-meaning-of-christmas-drops-19-k-on-cps-gifts

www.ingramcontent.com/pod-product-compliance
Lightning Source LLC
Chambersburg PA
CBHW052157110526
44591CB00012B/1984